CORE CASES

CORE CASES IN OBSTETRIC ANAESTHESIA

Edited by

Paul Clyburn
Consultant Anaesthetist
University Hospital of Wales
Cardiff

Rachel Collis
Consultant Anaesthetist
University Hospital of Wales
Cardiff

Mike Harmer
Head of Department of Anaesthetics
and Intensive Care Medicine
University of Wales College of
Medicine Cardiff

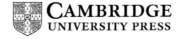

CAMBRIDGE
UNIVERSITY PRESS

CAMBRIDGE UNIVERISTY PRESS

Cambridge, New York, Melbourne, Madrid, Cape Town, Singapore, São Paulo, Delhi

Cambridge University Press
The Edinburgh Building, Cambridge CB2 8RU, UK

Published in the United States of America by Cambridge University Press, New York

www.cambridge.org
Information on this title: www.cambridge.org/9781841101606

© Greenwich Medical Media 2004

First published 2004
Reprinted by Cambridge University Press 2008

Printed in the United Kingdom at the University Press, Cambridge

ISBN 978-1841-10160-6 paperback

CONTENTS

PREFACE

There was once a time when learning was a simple matter of reading a standard large textbook on the desired topic and following the instructions. The problem with such an approach has always been the impersonality of the delivery of such information and often difficulty in placing such in the clinical setting. One way round this has been the development of a problem-based learning approach where the process centres on a specific topic and allows the student to explore relevant information both in depth and in breadth. Experience would also suggest that successful learning can be achieved by the individual patient teaching approach; the major benefit of this being that any problem is covered in a patient-orientated manner with scope for a holistic approach to management.

This book seeks to build on such an approach whereby a specific obstetric anaesthetic problem is discussed in a clinical setting. The topics chosen are mainly everyday situations that can cause problems in management. For each case, the text aims to identify the problem, outline the pathophysiology involved and discuss a management strategy. Each case is deliberately kept short to allow the reader to 'dip in' whenever they have a few spare minutes. It is not intended to be read from cover to cover but sampled in an order that appeals. Neither is it intended as a comprehensive text on obstetric anaesthesia but more as a 'sampler' of possible topics.

The authors are all members of the South Wales Obstetric Anaesthetists Forum and are involved in the day-to-day care of mothers. Thus we hope the advice proffered is both authoritative and relevant. We hope that you will both enjoy reading this small book and learn some useful lessons in specific areas.

Paul Clyburn
Rachel Collis
Mike Harmer

October 2003

CONTRIBUTORS

Andrew Bagwell *Specialist Registrar, Welsh School of Anaesthesia, Wales*

Chantal Busby *Consultant Anaesthetist, Princess of Wales Hospital, Bridgend*

Christopher C. Callander *Consultant Anaesthetist, Royal Gwent Hospital, Newport*

Alison Carling *Consultant Anaesthetist, Royal Gwent Hospital, Newport*

Susan Catling *Consultant Obstetric Anaesthetist, Singleton Hospital, Swansea*

Paul Clyburn *Consultant Anaesthetist, University Hospital of Wales, Cardiff*

Rachel Collis *Consultant Anaesthetist, University Hospital of Wales, Cardiff*

Jill Curtis *Consultant Anaesthetist, Royal Gwent Hospital, Newport*

J.S. Stuart Davies *Consultant Anaesthetist, Singleton Hospital, Swansea*

Christian Egeler *Consultant Anaesthetist, Singleton Hospital, Swansea*

Katherine A. Eggers *Consultant Anaesthetist, Princess of Wales Hospital, Bridgend*

Moira J. Evans *Consultant Anaesthetist, Singleton Hospital, Swansea*

Claire Farley *Specialist Registrar, Welsh School of Anaesthesia, Wales*

Oscar Fredy *Specialist Registrar, Mersey School of Anaesthesia, Liverpool*

Alison C. Garrard *Specialist Registrar, Welsh School of Anaesthesia, Wales*

Jonathan Griffiths *Consultant Anaesthetist, Royal Gwent Hospital, Newport*

Michael Harmer *Professor and Head of Academic Department of Anaesthetics and Intensive Care Medicine, University of Wales College of Medicine, Cardiff*

Christopher P.H. Heneghan *Consultant Anaesthetist, Nevill Hall Hospital, Abergavenny*

John C. Hughes *Consultant Anaesthetist, Princess of Wales Hospital, Bridgend*

Susan Jeffs *Consultant Anaesthetist, Nevill Hall Hospital, Abergavenny*

Melanie J.T. Jones *Consultant Anaesthetist, Princess of Wales Hospital, Bridgend*

S.K. Krishnan *Specialist Registrar, Welsh School of Anaesthesia, Wales*

Sarah Lloyd Jones *Locum Consultant Anaesthetist, Royal Gwent Hospital, Newport*

Cyprien Mendonca *Consultant Anaesthetist, Walsgrave Hospital, Coventry*

Gareth Parry *Specialist Registrar, Welsh School of Anaesthesia, Wales*

John Sewell *Consultant Anaesthetist, Royal Glamorgan Hospital, Llantrisant*

Mark Stacey *Consultant Anaesthetist, Llandough Hospital, Cardiff*

P.S. Sudheer *Lecturer in Anaesthesia, University of Wales College of Anaesthetists, Cardiff*

1

ANTICOAGULATION AND REGIONAL ANAESTHESIA

A.C. Garrard and M. Stacey

CASE HISTORY

A 32-year-old, gravida 5, para 0 woman suffering from myotonic dystrophy was admitted to hospital at 30 weeks gestation with raised blood pressure and oedema. Previously, the patient had suffered multiple miscarriages. For this reason, she had been taking aspirin (75 mg daily) and subcutaneous injections of enoxaparin (20 mg daily) throughout the pregnancy. Investigations revealed that she was homozygous for the Leiden mutation in the factor V gene.

The diagnosis of myotonic dystrophy had been made by a neurologist a year previously and confirmed by electromyography and muscle biopsy. During this pregnancy, her myotonia had worsened. She was able to walk only very short distances and on two occasions she was admitted to hospital with chest infections. Her only previous anaesthetic was uneventful and several years prior to her diagnosis.

On this admission, her blood pressure was initially 140/100 mmHg. She had marked oedema of her hands and feet, and mild proteinuria. She had no headache, visual disturbance or abdominal pain. Her blood pressure settled soon after admission and she was started on betamethasone. The following day, she complained of blurred vision and headache and her blood pressure had risen to 165/108 mmHg. Following a fluid preload, she received a bolus of hydralazine 5 mg, followed by an infusion at 2 mg/h. Her blood pressure again settled and the infusion was discontinued.

On examination, she had myotonic facies with frontal balding and bilateral ptosis. There was marked wasting of her neck and shoulder muscles. Examination of the respiratory system revealed decreased chest expansion but was otherwise unremarkable. Blood pressure was now stable at 140/90 mmHg and examination of the cardiovascular system was unremarkable. Fluid balance was +2300 ml for the previous 24 h. On examining her airway, she had full dentition, a slightly receding jaw and was assessed to be Mallampati class 2. Investigations are summarised in Table 1.1.

A decision was made to perform urgent Caesarean section the following morning. No further doses of enoxaparin were given. Ranitidine 150 mg was administered that night and again the following morning. In the anaesthetic room, full monitoring was established and an intravenous infusion of Hartmann's solution 1000 ml with ephedrine 30 mg was started. Uneventful spinal anaesthesia was performed at the L4/L5 interspace with 2.4 ml hyperbaric bupivacaine 0.5%, fentanyl 15 µg and morphine 100 µg. The patient was placed supine with a left lateral tilt. An adequate anaesthetic block was established (T4 to ice, T6 to touch). Following delivery of a healthy boy, syntocinon 5 IU was given and surgery completed uneventfully with a total blood loss of 500 ml. Postoperatively, the patient was monitored on the high dependency unit (HDU), with close attention to her respiratory rate. Analgesia was provided with rectal diclofenac and regular paracetamol.

DEFINITION OF THE PROBLEM

Spinal haematoma is an uncommon but serious complication of spinal or epidural anaesthesia, with patients receiving anticoagulants being at greater risk. The issue has become more important with the increased use of low-molecular-weight-heparin (LMWH) in the treatment and prevention of venous thrombo-embolic disease.

Table 1.1 – Investigations.

Haematology		Arterial blood gases	
Hb	11.0 g/dl	pH	7.41
WBC	$9.3 \times 10^9/l$	PaO_2	10.8 kPa
Platelets	$257 \times 10^9/l$	$PaCO_2$	4.5 kPa
Coagulation		Pulmonary function tests	
Fibrinogen	2.2 g/l	FEV_1	1.4 l
PT	9.7 s	FVC	1.8 l
APTT	27.1 s	FEV_1/FVC	78%
Biochemistry		Echocardiography within	
Na^+	134 mmol/l	normal limits	
K^+	4.1 mmol/l	12-lead ECG unremarkable	
Urea	2.2 mmol/l	Chest X-ray – lungs clear	
Creatinine	60 µmol/l		
Urate	0.41 mmol/l		
LFT	normal		

Myotonic dystrophy is an uncommon genetic condition. General anaesthesia exposes affected patients to risk and regional anaesthesia is safer.

PATHOPHYSIOLOGY

Myotonic dystrophy

This is an autosomal-dominant condition affecting skeletal, cardiac and smooth muscles. Patients usually present aged 20–40 years and die in their sixth decade from cardiac disease or bulbar muscle involvement. Myotonia is precipitated by cold, shivering, hyperkalaemia, suxamethonium and neostigmine. Neither regional nor general anaesthesia prevents myotonia as it is a primary myopathy. Patients with myotonic dystrophy have increased sensitivity to anaesthetic drugs and opiates. Suxamethonium is contraindicated as myotonic spasm may make intubation and ventilation impossible.

There is also increased sensitivity to non-depolarising neuromuscular-blocking drugs. A period of postoperative ventilation is often required following general anaesthesia due to decreased respiratory reserve. In addition, there is an increased incidence of difficult intubation and of regurgitation and pulmonary aspiration due to bulbar muscle weakness and decreased oesophageal tone. For these reasons, a regional technique was felt to be preferable to general anaesthesia.

Factor V Leiden

The factor V Leiden mutation causes resistance to the anticoagulant activity of activated protein C and is present in about 5% of Northern European individuals. There is an association between factor V Leiden and hypertensive disorders of pregnancy, first- and second-trimester miscarriage, placental infarction and placental abruption. The risk of venous thrombo-embolism in pregnancy rises from 1 in 1500 in the normal population to 4% for those homozygous for the Leiden mutation. Although LMWH is not thought to be indicated during pregnancy in these patients, it should be considered post-partum, particularly after operative delivery. This patient, however, was taking LMWH as treatment for recurrent miscarriage. Although it was thought that the benefits of a regional technique outweighed the risks, the danger of subarachnoid or epidural haematoma had to be considered.

MANAGEMENT OPTIONS AND DISCUSSION

Incidence of spinal haematoma

Spinal haematoma is a rare event and, therefore, large numbers of patients have to be studied in order to assess its incidence and predisposing risk factors. For this reason, prospective studies are difficult and most studies are based on retrospective analysis of case reports. A further complicating factor is that spinal haematoma can occur spontaneously in patients who have not received a spinal/epidural block, or do not have a coagulation defect. Epidural bleeding is more common than sub-arachnoid bleeding because of the prominent epidural venous plexus. Bleeding is least likely to become clinically significant in the intrathecal space, presumably because of the diluting effect of the cerebrospinal fluid (CSF). The estimated incidence of spinal haematoma following epidural procedures is estimated to be less than 1 in 150,000 and less than 1 in 220,000 after spinal block.

Risk factors

Vandermeulen in a literature search extending back to 1906, found 61 cases of spinal haematoma associated with spinal or epidural anaesthesia (see Further reading, Horlocker and Wedel (1998)); 42 of these patients had received anticoagulant drugs, had a clotting disorder, or were thrombocytopenic. Full therapeutic anti-coagulation with either warfarin or intravenous heparin is accepted as a contraindication to central neural blockade. The position regarding low-dose anticoagulants is less clear. Vandermeulen found that prophylaxis with low-dose unfractionated heparin (LDUH) was rarely associated with spinal bleeding complications. However, the use of LMWH has been associated with an increased risk of spinal haematoma.

Non-steroidal anti-inflammatory drugs (NSAIDs) when used alone are not a significant risk factor in the development of spinal haematoma. Aspirin therapy inhibits platelet aggregation and ideally should be stopped 7–10 days before the spinal or epidural procedures. However, this may be contraindicated in patients taking aspirin for certain conditions, such as carotid artery stenosis. It should also be noted that in the Collaborative Low-Dose Aspirin Study (CLASP study), many obstetric patients received aspirin and epidural analgesia without complication. However, the combined use of aspirin, NSAIDs and LMWH with central neural blockade is thought to increase the risk of spinal bleeding and should be avoided.

In the study by Vandermeulen, needle placement was difficult in 25% patients and multiple punctures were reported in a further 20%. Bloody taps were noted in 10–40% of cases, and some authors believe this to be a contraindication to anti-coagulation. In the majority of cases, more than one risk factor was present. Insertion and removal of catheters was shown to have a strong association with spinal haematoma, with a lower incidence if a single-shot technique was used. Abnormal anatomy of the back (causing difficult needle placement), anatomical abnormalities (e.g. spina bifida occulta), vascular abnormalities and spinal stenosis (also causing difficult insertion) have been identified as risk factors.

Low-molecular-weight heparin

LMWHs are linear polysaccharides prepared by fractionating standard heparin and separating out the shorter chain fragments with molecular weights of between 4000 and 6000 Da. Both unfractionated heparin and LMWHs exert their anti-coagulant activity by binding to anti-thrombin via a pentasaccharide sequence. This induces a conformational change, which allows anti-thrombin to bind factor Xa and thrombin, and inactivate them. The shorter chain length of LMWH allows binding to only Xa, while unfractionated heparin will bind both Xa and thrombin (see Figure 1.1). Thus, LMWH allows a selective inhibition of factor Xa (see Figure 1.2 for a summary of the coagulation cascade).

LMWHs produce a more predictable anticoagulant effect than unfractionated heparin, with better bioavailability and dose-independent clearance. The plasma half-life is two to four times as long as that of unfractionated heparin, ranging from 3 to 6 h after subcutaneous injection. Therefore, it needs to be given only once or twice a day. Due to the more predictable response, monitoring is often not required, although assays of anti-Xa activity do provide reliable information about the anti-thrombotic effect of LMWHs. Activated partial thromboplastin time (APTT) accurately reflects the anti-haemostatic potential of unfractionated heparin but bears little or no resemblance to that of LMWHs. This is because LMWHs

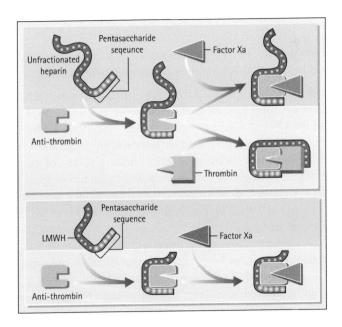

Figure 1.1 – Catalysis of anti-thrombin-mediated inactivation of thrombin or factor Xa by unfractionated heparin or LMWHs. The interaction of unfractionated heparin and LMWHs with anti-thrombin is mediated by the pentasaccharide sequence of the drugs. Binding of either to anti-thrombin causes a conformational change at its reactive centre that accelerates its interaction with factor Xa. Consequently, both unfractionated heparin and LMWHs catalyse the inactivation of factor Xa by anti-thrombin. In contrast to factor Xa inhibition, catalysis of anti-thrombin-mediated inactivation of thrombin requires the formation of a ternary heparin–anti-thrombin–thrombin complex. This complex can be formed only by chains at least 18-saccharide units long. This explains why LMWHs have less inhibitory activity against thrombin than unfractionated heparin. Reproduced with permission from Weitz JI. Low molecular weight repairs. *The New England Journal of Medicine* 1997; **337**: 688–98. ©*1997 Massachussetts Medical Society. All rights reserved.*

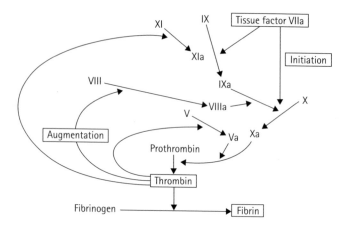

Figure 1.2 – The coagulation cascade. Reproduced with permission from Vickers, Morgan, Spenser, Read. *Drugs in Anaesthesia Intensive Care Practice*, 8th edn. Butterworth Heinemann 1999.

catalyse thrombin inhibition by anti-thrombin to a much lesser extent. Unlike unfractionated heparin, LMWHs cannot be reversed by protamine.

The estimated incidence of spinal haematoma in European patients treated with enoxaparin and neuroaxial block is extremely low at 1 in 2,250,000. However, experience in the USA is quite different. Up until June 1998, the manufacturer of the USA brand of enoxaparin, Lovenox, had received more than 50 reports of patients developing spinal haematoma with concurrent use of enoxaparin and neuroaxial block. In the light of these reports, the frequency of spinal haematoma in USA patients receiving enoxaparin after spinal or epidural anaesthesia was estimated to be nearer 1 in 1000. This discrepancy between European and USA experience may be explained by the difference in dosing between the continents (30 mg twice daily in the USA, as compared with 40 mg once daily in Europe). As a result of these reports, it has been suggested that the dose of enoxaparin should not exceed 40 mg daily, that central neural blockade or removal of an epidural catheter should be delayed by at least 12 h following LMWH, and that the next dose should then not be given for a further 2 h.

Monitoring, diagnosis and treatment of spinal haematoma

The most common signs and symptoms of developing spinal haematoma and cord compression are leg weakness and sensory loss, urinary retention, back pain and paraplegia. Unfortunately, the presence of continuing central neural blockade with infusion of local anaesthetics makes recognition of these signs extremely difficult. Frequent observation by a trained individual is essential. If any suspicion exists, an urgent magnetic resonance imaging (MRI) scan or myelogram must be arranged. Outcome after spinal or epidural bleeding is frequently poor. However, up to 80% of patients can recover good spinal function if decompressive laminectomy is performed within 8 h. Decompression performed later than 24 h is generally associated with a poor outcome.

Although patients with myotonia are at increased risk of respiratory depression following the use of opiates, a small intrathecal dose was thought to be safe, with close monitoring postoperatively. An alternative technique would have been a combined spinal epidural, with hyperbaric bupivacaine alone as the intrathecal component, followed by an infusion of plain bupivacaine for postoperative analgesia. Although this would have avoided the use of opiates, it would have made postoperative neurological monitoring difficult.

KEY LEARNING POINTS

1. Full anticoagulation is a contraindication to central nervous blockade.

2. Patients with abnormal spinal anatomy may be more likely to develop spinal haematomas. Bloody taps and multiple or difficult punctures are also risk factors.

3. Patients on aspirin may have a central nervous block by a skilled operator, if followed by careful neurological monitoring.

4. Perioperative prophylaxis by LDUH or LMWH should be delayed and given after central nervous blockade.

5. The dose of enoxaparin should be limited to 40 mg daily. High-dose treatment for proven venous thrombo-embolic disease is a contraindication to central nervous blockade.

6. Where LMWH has been given, central nervous blockade should be delayed by 12 h. After LDUH wait 4–6 h.

7. The combination of LMWH and aspirin plus NSAIDs increases the risk of intraspinal bleeding.

8. Catheter removal should be delayed until 12 h after LMWH administration and 4 h after LDUH.

9. Following central neural blockade or removal of an epidural catheter, a simple system of regular neurological monitoring should be instituted and followed by trained staff.

10. If there is any suspicion of spinal haematoma an urgent MRI scan must be performed.

11. Urgent neurosurgical decompression should be arranged within 8 h if a spinal haematoma is diagnosed.

Further reading

Armstrong RF, Addy V, Brevik H. Epidural and spinal anaesthesia and the use of anticoagulants. *Hospital Medicine* 1999; **60**: 491–6.

Bergquist D, Lindblad B, Matzsch T. Risk of combining low molecular weight heparin for thromboprophylaxis and epidural or spinal anaesthesia. *Seminars in Thrombosis and Hemostasis* 1993; **19** (suppl. 1): 147–51.

Bullingham A, Strunin L. Prevention of venous thromboembolism. *British Journal of Anaesthesia* 1995; **75**: 622–30.

Campbell A, Thompson N. Anaesthesia for caesarean section in a patient with myotonic dystrophy receiving warfarin therapy. *Canadian Journal of Anaesthesia* 1995; **42**: 409–14.

Dolenska S. Neuroaxial blocks and LMWH thromboprophylaxis. *Hospital Medicine* 1998; **59**: 940–3.

Horlocker TT. Low molecular weight heparins. *New England Journal of Medicine* 1998; **338**: 687.

Horlocker TT, Wedel DJ. Spinal and epidural blockade and perioperative low molecular weight heparin: smooth sailing on the Titanic. *Anesthesia and Analgesia* 1998; **86**: 1153–6.

Horlocker TT, Wedel DJ, Schroeder DR, *et al*. Preoperative antiplatelet therapy does not increase the risk of spinal haematoma associated with regional anaesthesia. *Anesthesia and Analgesia* 1995; **80**: 303–9.

Rolbin SH, Abbot D, Musclow D, Papsin F, Lie LM, Freedman J. Epidural anaesthesia in pregnant patients with low platelet counts. *Obstetrics and Gynaecology* 1988; **71**: 394–5.

Tryba M. Epidural regional anaesthesia and low molecular weight heparin. *Pro (German) Anesth Intensivmed Notfallmed Schmerzther* 1993; **28**: 179–81.

Tryba M, Wedel DJ. Central neuraxial block and low molecular heparin (enoxaparin): lessons learned from different dosage regimes in two continents. *Acta Anaesthesiologica Scandinavica* 1997; **41** (suppl. 1): 100–3.

Vandermeulen EP, Van Aken H, Vermylen J. Anticoagulants and spinal–epidural anaesthesia. *Anesthesia and Analgesia* 1994; **79**: 1165–77.

Weitz JI. Low molecular weight heparins. *The New England Journal of Medicine* 1997; **337**: 688–98.

Wulf H. Epidural anaesthesia and spinal haematoma. *Canadian Journal of Anaesthesia* 1996; **43**: 1260–71.

2

ASTHMA DURING PREGNANCY

G. Parry and M.J.T. Jones

CASE HISTORY

A 29-year-old primigravida of 30 weeks gestation presented to the accident and emergency department with dyspnoea.

She had a past medical history of asthma, which was normally well controlled on inhaled beclomethasone dipropionate 200 mg bd and inhaled salbutamol prn. Since learning of her pregnancy, she had stopped taking the inhaled steroid.

Over the previous 2 months, she had felt a little short of breath and had been using increased doses of salbutamol. For 2 days, she had felt generally unwell with increasing dyspnoea, which was unrelieved by her salbutamol. She eventually presented to the accident and emergency department at 8 p.m.

On examination, she looked comfortable, was alert and talking in short sentences. Her pulse rate was 100 beats/min and regular, and blood pressure 130/80 mmHg. Her respiratory rate was 28 breaths/min, oxygen saturation (by pulse oximetry [SpO_2]) 98% on 6 l/min of oxygen via a face mask, peak-expiratory flow rate (PEFR) was 250 l/min, and there was widespread wheeze throughout the chest. Her initial blood gases are shown in Table 2.1 (Sample 1).

The patient was treated with nebulised salbutamol 5 mg and budesonide 1 mg (she refused oral steroids), there was marginal improvement, and she was admitted to a general medical ward at 10 p.m. for regular nebulised therapy.

Over the following 8 h, there was a marked deterioration and by 6 a.m. she was in extremis. She was drowsy and unable to speak, her respiratory rate was 60 breaths/min, SpO_2 85% on 15 l/min of oxygen by face mask, and chest auscultation was almost silent. Her pulse was 68 beats/min and blood pressure 95/60 mmHg. She was urgently referred to intensive care, and on the arrival of the anaesthetist, further blood-gas results were available (Table 2.1, Sample 2).

With the help of a skilled assistant, the anaesthetist placed the mother supine in the left-tilted position. She was pre-oxygenated with 100% oxygen via a tight-fitting face mask, cricoid pressure was applied and she was anaesthetised with ketamine 200 mg and suxamethonium 100 mg, and her trachea was intubated. Neuromuscular paralysis was maintained with vecuronium 8 mg and she was transferred to the intensive care ward, intubated and ventilated.

During transfer, she was very difficult to ventilate and she was commenced on intravenous salbutamol $0.5 \mu g/kg/min$, a loading dose of aminophylline $5 \mu g/kg$ over 30 min, followed by an infusion $0.5 \mu g/kg/h$ and hydrocortisone 100 mg 6-hourly. Arterial and central venous access was established on arrival in the intensive care unit, and a nasogastric tube was passed, through which she was given antacid therapy.

She was ventilated using a time-cycled, pressure-controlled mode, with a respiratory rate of 10, peak pressure of $40 \, cmH_2O$, I : E ratio of 1 : 3.5, and no positive end-expiratory pressure (PEEP). This achieved a SpO_2 of 98%, but a minute volume of only 4 l and, at this time, mediastinal air was noted on her chest X-ray. She was sedated with propofol and alfentanil, and neuromuscular paralysis was continued with vecuronium. Blood gases were repeated (Table 2.1, Sample 3).

Tidal volumes were still small, and halothane at 0.6% was introduced into the breathing circuit; after 4 h, the tidal volume had started to increase and there was improvement in the blood gases (Table 2.1, Sample 4).

A cardiotocogram (CTG) was commenced and the obstetrician reviewed the patient's pregnancy and in discussion with the neonatologist, the opinion was to continue the pregnancy if her pH was >7.2, SpO_2 > 94%, and the CTG remained favourable.

There was gradual improvement over the next few hours. Blood was taken for an aminophylline level at 4 p.m., which was found to be satisfactory. The halothane was stopped by 12 h and the minute volume had increased to 7 l by 24 h (Table 2.1, Sample 5). By 48 h, a minute volume of 8.5 l had been achieved, neuromuscular blockers were stopped, and the peak pressure was reduced (Table 2.1, Sample 6). Intravenous salbutamol was changed to inhaled salbutamol via the breathing system, and 12 h later, sedative drugs were discontinued and the patient was extubated successfully.

> The patient spent 2 more days on the intensive care unit before being transferred to a ward, the aminophylline was weaned off, and prednisolone replaced hydrocortisone. She was discharged from hospital 5 days later.
>
> At 39 weeks, she went into spontaneous labour and with epidural analgesia, had an uneventful delivery of a healthy baby boy.

DESCRIPTION OF THE PROBLEM

- Physiological changes in pregnancy are usually well tolerated; they can, however, lead to dyspnoea in women with no respiratory disease.

- Asthma is the most common respiratory disease in women of child-bearing age, and can be exacerbated by pregnancy.

- The severity of the attack may not be recognised.

- Exacerbations may be related to discontinuation of maintenance medication or respiratory infection.

PATHOPHYSIOLOGY

Pregnancy results in many changes in respiratory physiology. Increased progesterone results in an increase in minute volume by 40–50%. The tidal volume increases significantly more than the respiratory rate, which may remain unchanged. Oxygen consumption increases by 20–30% and carbon dioxide production increases, but proportionately less than the increase in alveolar ventilation. This results in a decrease in the partial pressure of arterial CO_2 to approximately 3.6–4.2 kPa, and a mild respiratory alkalosis, although an increased renal excretion of bicarbonate prevents a further rise in pH. Functional residual capacity decreases by 20% by term

Table 2.1 – Blood gas analysis of study patient.

	Blood gases (samples)					
	1: At presentation	2: Pre-intubation	3: Post-intubation	4: 4 h	5: 24 h	6: 48 h
pH	7.39	7.04	7.09	7.2	7.30	7.38
$PaCO_2$ (kPa)	5	12.1	13.4	9.2	7.2	4.2
PaO_2 (kPa)	14	6.3	15.4	18.6	15.5	16.2
Standard bicarbonate (mmol/l)	24	12	14	17	20	22
Base excess (mmol/l)	3	−8	−7	−3	0	1
SaO_2 (percentage)	98	83	97	98	98	99

but PEFR remains unchanged during the course of pregnancy. These changes are usually well tolerated, but up to 75% of women complain of dyspnoea at some time during pregnancy.

Asthma is characterised by inflammation and swelling of respiratory mucosa; bronchiolar muscle hyper-reactivity and spasm; and mucous plugging of small airways. These changes result in increased airway resistance and reduced flow in the airways. Asthma complicates approximately 1–4% of pregnancies and the incidence appears to be rising, possibly due to increased recognition. Asthma continues to be associated with a significant morbidity and mortality. The common problems are non-compliance with treatment and severity that is underestimated by patients and doctors.

Assessment of the severity of asthma is based largely on history, examination findings and PEFR (Table 2.2). Arterial blood-gas analysis is also helpful (Table 2.3). Chest radiograph should not be withheld if indicated, the dose of ionising radiation is less than $\frac{1}{20}$ th of the safe maximum during pregnancy.

Approximately 25% of women report a deterioration of their asthma during pregnancy; the peak of symptoms is at 28–36 weeks gestation. Most women improve during the last 4 weeks of pregnancy, and exacerbations during parturition are rare. Predicting which patients will deteriorate is difficult. There is evidence that those patients with the most severe asthma are more likely to deteriorate, as are those women whose symptoms increased in previous pregnancies.

Asthma in pregnancy has been associated with maternal and foetal complications. Pregnancy-induced hypertension and gestational diabetes are more common in women with severe asthma, possibly due to the effects of systemic corticosteroids.

Table 2.2 – British Thoracic Society: assessment of severity of asthma.

Potentially life threatening	Immediately life threatening
Unable to complete sentences	PEFR <33%
Respiratory rate >25	Silent chest, cyanosis, feeble respiratory effort
Pulse >110	Bradycardia or hypotension
PEFR <50% predicted or best	Exhaustion, confusion or coma
PEFR <200 l/min	
Arterial parodox >10 mmHg	

Table 2.3 – Blood-gas analysis in asthma.

Severity	PaO_2	$PaCO_2$	pH
Mild	N or ↓	N or ↓	N or ↑
Mild/moderate	↓	↓	↑
Moderate/severe	↓	N	N
Severe	↓↓	↑↑	↓↓

An increase in the incidence of ante- and post-partum haemorrhage has also been described. Low birth weight, intra-uterine growth retardation, and an increased incidence of premature birth are all recognised complications and there is an association with neonatal hyperbilirubinaemia, and an increase in intra-uterine and perinatal deaths in babies of women with asthma.

MANAGEMENT OPTIONS AND DISCUSSION

Close monitoring and a multidisciplinary approach with good communication between physician, obstetrician, neonatoligist and anaesthetist are essential.

When asthma is severe, the aims of treatment are: to prevent maternal death, respiratory failure and episodes of status asthmaticus, and to improve maternal symptoms, as well as not compromising the growth or maturation of the foetus. With aggressive therapy, these goals can be achieved, and the outcome of pregnancy, even in steroid-dependent women, approaches that of the general population.

Broadly speaking, the treatment of asthma in pregnancy is no different to the non-pregnant state. The risk to the mother and foetus from undertreatment is greater than any effect of commonly used asthma medications on the foetus.

Oxygen

Early administration of oxygen is essential. One of the principle aims of treatment is to prevent maternal and foetal hypoxia. Initially, as the maternal partial pressure of arterial oxygen (PaO_2) decreases there is little change in oxygen content, however, the foetal oxy-haemoglobin dissociation curve is such that a small fall in foetal PaO_2 results in a large decrease in oxygen content.

Maternal hyperventilation results in an alkalosis, and a shift of the oxy-haemoglobin dissociation curve to the left, resulting in a decreased oxygen transfer to the foetus. Alkalosis also causes the uterine vasculature to constrict, and possibly causes increased intraplacental shunting, further diminishing oxygen delivery to the foetus.

Maternal acidosis results in a shift in the oxy-haemaglobin dissociation curve in favour of the foetus. In this severe state, however, the increase in endogenous catacholamines results in uterine artery vasoconstriction and reduced oxygen delivery to the foetus. These changes make it essential to maintain the maternal PaO_2 as near normal as possible.

β_2-Agonists

When inhaled, only small quantities of β_2-agonists reach the systemic circulation. This is the preferred route of administration and there is considerable experience in the use of salbutamol and terbutaline during pregnancy, which are considered safe. There is growing experience in pregnancy with the longer-acting β_2-agonists and they are also considered safe. If indicated, intravenous β_2-agonists should not be withheld, although tachycardia may limit the dose.

Tocolytic therapy with the β_2-agonists salbutamol and terbutaline has been associated with maternal pulmonary odema, the pathophysiology of which remains obscure, and although not directly linked with asthma treatment, this potential side effect should be considered in pregnancy.

Corticosteroids

Of all anti-asthma medication, reluctance to prescribe corticosteroids is the most prevalent. This is based on an unfounded fear, as extensive experience in their use has failed to demonstrate any relationship between their use and congenital malformation. There is a small association between systemic corticosteroids in asthma and intra-uterine growth retardation, reflecting the effect of severe asthma on foetal growth, rather than an effect of the drug. Evidence suggests that episodes of severe asthma are more risk to the foetus than treatment with corticosteroids and avoidance of attacks is essential for foetal well-being.

The most experience is with inhaled beclomethasone dipropionate, which is considered to be safe, and although there is less experience with budesonide, it is also thought to be safe.

Women taking systemic corticosteroids are at increased risk of pregnancy-induced hypertension and gestational diabetes. However, systemic corticosteroids may be essential to control symptoms, or even life saving when used to treat status asthmaticus. Prednisolone is extensively metabolised by the placenta, and levels in the foetus only reach 10% of maternal levels; it is the systemic corticosteroid of choice during pregnancy. Foetal levels approach 30% of maternal with hydrocortisone but it should still be used in the emergency situation.

Steroids take several hours to be effective, and systemic corticosteroids should be given early, and in sufficient doses to prevent excessive risk to mother and foetus.

Methyl xanthines

Xanthines readily cross the placenta and foetal levels are similar to maternal; however, there is no conclusive evidence of any ill effect. Transient irritability and tachycardia have been noted in neonates of mothers on theophylline, but it is considered safe to use during pregnancy as third-line therapy for asthma. Pharmacokinetics are altered in pregnancy, with increased volume of distribution, decreased protein binding and decreased clearance, especially during the third trimester. Levels should be checked every 2–3 weeks during this time, aiming for a plasma level of 8–12 μg/ml.

Intravenous aminophylline is recommended for status asthmaticus, and the loading dose in pregnancy (if indicated) is not changed from the non-pregnant state.

More caution is required for the maintenance dose, and blood levels should be checked at 10–12 h.

Anticholinergics

Inhaled ipratropium bromide is considered safe in pregnancy.

Mechanical ventilation

Occasionally, the patient fails to improve, or deteriorates and needs mechanical ventilation despite maximal medical therapy. The indications for ventilation are no different to the non-pregnant state, namely exhaustion, feeble respiratory effort, decreased level of consciousness, deteriorating PEFR, deteriorating or persisting hypoxia, hypercapnia or respiratory arrest.

Arterial oxygenation will decrease rapidly on induction of anaesthesia. Pre-oxygenation with 100% oxygen is essential. Cricoid pressure should be used to prevent aspiration of stomach contents in pregnant patients. Cardiovascular instability at induction of anaesthesia will be more pronounced because of aorto-caval compression and a lateral tilt or manual displacement of the uterus should be employed.

Ketamine causes an increase in sympathetic tone, preserving heart rate and blood pressure. Bronchodilation and prevention of bronchospasm are also characteristic features and for these reasons, it is the induction agent of choice in this situation.

The initial ventilation strategy is to prevent hypoxia, and allow the maximal time for expiration thus preventing air trapping, and minimising auto-PEEP:

- Maintenance of PaO_2 with a high percentage of inspired oxygen, if needed.

- Tidal volumes of <10 ml/kg.

- Rate <10 breaths/min, long I : E ratio $>1 : 2.5$, and peak inspiratory flow rate >80 l/min. These help to prolong the expiratory time.

- Peak airway pressure <40 cmH$_2$O, PEEP <5 cmH$_2$O.

These settings are likely to result in a mild respiratory acidosis initially, but permissive hypercarbia is acceptable if the pH is greater than 7.2. Airway resistance will alter significantly with disease severity and treatment. Ventilatory settings need frequent review and assessment, including arterial blood-gas sampling.

Neuromuscular block may be required, initially. This reduces peak airway pressures, may be essential to allow permissive hypercapnia, and reduces carbon dioxide production.

Inhalational anaesthetics

Inhalational anaesthetics cause relaxation of bronchial smooth muscle, but also cause respiratory and myocardial depression in a dose-dependent manner. In ventilated patients with life-threatening asthma, halothane has been recommended, in concentrations of 0.3–1.5%, to reverse bronchospasm. Rapid improvement of hypoxia, hypercapnia, acidosis and lung mechanics usually results in circulatory improvement. Ventricular dysrhythmias are well recognised in association with halothane; these can be exacerbated by ongoing sympathomimetic requirements or aminophylline toxicity, and isoflurane can be used as an alternative in these situations.

Other treatments

Extracorporeal membrane oxygenation has been described in asthma and during pregnancy, with good maternal and foetal outcome.

Termination of pregnancy during life-threatening asthma has also resulted in rapid improvement of lung mechanics.

Analgesia and anaesthesia for delivery

Mothers with mild or well-controlled asthma can choose the method of analgesia they prefer. Prolonged use of Entonox, however, will dry respiratory secretions and should be advised against where wheeze is associated with this problem.

Regional analgesia for labour should be advised, if the mother's asthma has been difficult to control as it will help to prevent the hyperventilation that is associated with the pain and anxiety of delivery.

General anaesthesia should be avoided, if possible to reduce the risk of an exacerbation of respiratory symptoms. The choice between the different regional techniques is more controversial. The high block that is required for Caesarean section may make it difficult for the breathless mother to lie down and cough. The height of the block must be accurately controlled to T4 and a technique where the anaesthetic wears off rapidly is ideal.

KEY LEARNING POINTS

1. Maternal and foetal outcome is improved with good control of maternal asthma and the mother must be encouraged to continue on her normal medication.

2. There should be a multidisciplinary approach.

3. PEFRs are reliable during pregnancy and pregnancy can cause worsening of asthma.

4. Treatment of asthma is broadly unchanged by pregnancy.

5. Most commonly used asthma medications are considered safe in pregnancy.

6. There should be early aggressive management of exacerbations.

7. Maternal oxygen administration improves foetal oxygenation.

8. Regional anaesthetic techniques are helpful for labour and delivery.

Further reading

Alexander S, Dodds L, Armson BA. Perinatal outcomes in women with asthma during pregnancy. *Obstetrics and Gynecology* 1998; **92**: 435–40.

Brancazio LR, Laifer SA, Schwartz T. Peak expiratory flow rate in normal pregnancy. *Obstetrics and Gynecology* 1997; **89**: 383–6.

Cydulka RK, Emerman CL, Schreiber D, Molander KH, Woodruff PG, Camargo CA. Acute asthma among pregnant women presenting to the emergency department. *American Journal of Respiratory and Critical Care Medicine* 1999; **160**: 887–92.

Gelber M, Sidi Y, Gassner S, et al. Uncontrollable life-threatening status asthmaticus. An indication for termination of pregnancy by Caesarean section. *Respiration* 1987; **46**: 320–2.

Gluck JC, Gluck PA. The effects of pregnancy on asthma: a prospective study. *Annals of Allergy* 1976; **37**: 164–8.

Hollingsworth HM, Irwin RS. Acute respiratory failure in pregnancy. *Clinics in Chest Medicine* 1992; **13**: 723–40.

Kallen B, Rydhstroem H, Aberg A. Asthma during pregnancy – a population based study. *European Journal of Epidemiology* 2000; **16**: 167–71.

King PT, Rosalion A, McMillan J, Buist M, Holmes PW. Extracorporeal membrane oxygenation in pregnancy. *The Lancet* 2000; **356**: 45–6.

National Asthma Education Program. Report of the Working Group of Asthma and Pregnancy. Management of Asthma during Pregnancy. 1993, NIH publication 93-3279A.

Nelson-Piercy C, Morre-Gillon J. Asthma in pregnancy. *British Journal of Hospital Medicine* 1996; **55**: 115–17.

Rizk NW, Kalassian KG, Gilligan T, Druzin MI, Daniel DL. Obstetric complications in pulmonary and critical care medicine. *Chest* 1996; **110**: 791–809.

Rosseel P, Lauwers LF, Baute L. Halothane treatment in life-threatening asthma. *Intensive Care Medicine* 1985; **11**: 241–6.

Schatz M, Zeiger RS. Asthma and allergy in pregnancy. *Clinics in Perinatology* 1997; **24**: 407–32.

Schatz M, Zeiger RS, Hoffman C. Intrauterine growth is related to gestational pulmonary function in pregnant asthmatic women. *Chest* 1990; **98**: 389–92.

Schatz M, Zeiger RS, Harden K, Hoffman C, Chilingar L, Petitti D. The safety of asthma and allergy medications during pregnancy. *Journal of Allergy and Clinical Immunology* 1997; **100**: 301–6.

Schatz M, Harden K, Forsythe A, Chilingar L, Hoffman C, Sperling W, Zeiger RS. The course of asthma during pregnancy, post partum, and with successive pregnancies: a prospective analysis. *Journal of Allergy and Clinical Immunology* 1998; **81**: 509–16.

Schreier L, Cutler RM, Saigal V. Respiratory failure in asthma during the third trimester: report of two cases. *American Journal of Obstetrics and Gynecology* 1989; **160**: 80–1.

Shanies HM, Venkataraman MT, Peter T. Reversal of intractable acute severe asthma by first-trimester termination of pregnancy. *Journal of Asthma* 1997; **34**: 169–72.

Shnider SM, Levinson G. *Anaesthesia for Obstetrics.* Williams and Wilkins, Baltimore, 1993.

Thacker HL. Medical aspects of pregnancy. *Journal of Women's Health* 1999; **8**: 335–46.

The British Thoracic Society and others. Guidelines on the management of asthma. *Thorax* 1993; **48** (suppl.): S1–4.

The British Thoracic Society and others. The British guidelines on management of asthma. *Thorax* 1997; **52** (suppl.): S1–S21.

Turner ES, Greenberger PA, Patterson R. Management of the pregnant asthmatic patient. *Annals of Internal Medicine* 1980; **6**: 905–18.

Webb AR, Shipiro MJ, Singer M, Sater PM. *Oxford Textbook of Critical Care.* Oxford University Press, Oxford, 1999.

White RJ, Coutts I, Gibbs CJ, MacIntyre C. A prospective study of asthma during pregnancy and the puerperium. *Respiratory Medicine* 1989; **83**: 103–6.

3

BREECH DELIVERY

O. Fredy and R. Collis

CASE HISTORY

A slim, 24-year-old woman who had had a previous uncomplicated vaginal delivery with analgesia provided by an epidural, presented in active labour. On examination, she had a previously undiagnosed breech presentation with no evidence of a footling presentation, her cervix was 6 cm dilated, she was having strong contractions every 2 min and the presenting part was well within the pelvis at +1 to the ischial spines. Although she was coping well with the pain of her contractions using Entonox, she was giving involuntary pushes during her contractions because of the low presenting part. A cardiotocograph (CTG) was commenced, which confirmed foetal wellbeing with a baseline foetal heart rate of 145 beats/min with a good beat-to-beat variability and no decelerations.

In view of the uncomplicated breech presentation, her advancing labour and maternal wish, a plan for assisted breech delivery was made. Intravenous (IV) access was obtained with a 16G cannula. A combined spinal–epidural (CSE) procedure was performed to provide analgesia. The mother was placed in the sitting position and the epidural space at the L3–4 level was identified at 4.5 cm depth with a 16G-Tuohy needle. A 27G-Whitacre needle without stillette was introduced through the Tuohy needle and a flashback of clear cerebrospinal fluid (CSF) was seen. A 1 ml bolus of 0.25% bupivacaine (2.5 mg) with fentanyl 15 μg was given intrathecally. The spinal needle was removed and an epidural catheter threaded and fixed at the 9 cm mark to the skin.

Onset of analgesia was rapid and the patient was comfortable within 5 min. Sensory block to ice was up to T8 bilaterally and her urge to bear down diminished. She had little motor block and could perform a straight leg raise. The patient was advised to be as upright as possible and she chose to sit on a stool next to her bed, so that continuous CTG monitoring could continue. Analgesia was administered via the epidural catheter at 45–60 min intervals, using 10 ml of 0.1% bupivacaine with 0.0002% fentanyl solution.

Three hours after her CSE, she was examined and her cervix was fully dilated. The mother was comfortable throughout with little or no urge to bear down, she remained mobile and the foetal heart sounds were normal.

She was given an epidural top-up of 15 ml of the low-dose epidural solution at the start of the second stage of labour and was encouraged not to push until the presenting part was visible at the vulva. The mother had little perineal sensation of pain or stretching but felt an urge to bear down with contractions. After 30 min of active pushing, the breech was delivered spontaneously up to the umbilicus. An episiotomy was performed at this stage, and the shoulders delivered by gentle traction and the head by the Mariceau Smellie Veit manoeuvre. The mother had adequate analgesia for all the assisted manoeuvres and episiotomy suturing. The epidural catheter was removed at the end of the delivery.

A term female baby weighing 3.1 kg was delivered with Apgar scores of 7 and 9 at 1 and 5 min, respectively. The pH of the venous and arterial cord samples was 7.26 and 7.21, respectively.

DESCRIPTION OF THE PROBLEM

The incidence of breech presentation at term is 2.6–4%. With the possibility of a breech presentation in every 25 mothers, it is not surprising to find an undiagnosed breech in labour.

There has been a move away from vaginal breech delivery for some years and this attitude has been affirmed since the Term breech study, which showed that it was safer for the baby if delivered by Caesarean section:

1. There will be still some mothers who wish to attempt a vaginal delivery with a diagnosed breech.

2. Some women will present in labour with an undiagnosed breech.

It is, therefore, important not to lose all the skills associated with the safe vaginal delivery of the breech baby and to provide adequate analgesia to the mother, if she wishes it:

1. The safe delivery of the breech baby requires that the mother should be able to give maximal effort in bearing down, as it is dangerous to pull on the body of the breech for slow progress.

2. The mother needs appropriate analgesia for the assisted delivery of the head, especially when an episiotomy is performed.

MANAGEMENT OPTIONS AND DISCUSSION

Current obstetric practice advocates Caesarean section for any breech. Perinatal mortality, neonatal mortality and serious neonatal morbidity are relatively lower with Caesarean section when compared with a vaginal breech delivery. Serious maternal mortality and morbidity are understandably higher with Caesarean section, so some may argue that with an uncomplicated breech, a vaginal delivery is acceptable. The consensus is that planned Caesarean is safer when the breech presentation is a footling, when the foetus is compromised, premature, large or has congenital anomalies. Apart from the foetal factors, maternal factors like placenta praevia, inadequate liquor or foeto-pelvic disproportion could compromise a safe vaginal delivery.

The uncomplicated breech presentation, advanced labour and previous history of normal vaginal delivery are the factors that prompted a vaginal delivery in the above case.

If the breech presentation is diagnosed either in the antenatal period or in very early labour, then external cephalic version (ECV) can be attempted. It is usually attempted at 37 weeks, when there is adequate foetal lung maturity, thus avoiding the problems of a breech delivery. Reports of increased perinatal mortality are associated with this procedure and some obstetricians do not favour this approach.

Analgesia in the first stage of labour

In a breech presentation, the engaging bitrochanteric diameter is smaller than the engaging (suboccipito-frontal) diameter of the after-coming head. The small, soft and compliant breech leads the way and makes a track for the large, firm and less compliant head. In between the breech and the head lie the limbs, the trunk and the umbilical cord. Expediate delivery or obstructed passage to one or other parts leads to the possibility of complications. Sequential events of labour, an active labour mechanism and optimal anatomy are absolute essentials for a safe vaginal delivery.

The urge to bear down during the first stage, as in this case, may result in premature delivery of the breech through an incompletely dilated cervix. The resulting obstruction to the after-coming head leads to severe foetal morbidity or mortality. Hence the objectives of anaesthesia in the first stage are as follows:

1. good analgesia with good sacral spread,

2. adequate pelvic muscle tone,

3. motor power to aid mobility and pushing when required,

4. minimal foetal effects.

Regional techniques, either low-dose epidural or low-dose CSE analgesia, are ideal; other modes of systemic and inhalation analgesics do not provide the required effects.

A low-dose CSE was used in this case to establish analgesia rapidly and abolish the mother's urge to bear down. The even spread of the drug in the intrathecal fluid provides a uniform sensory block and minimal motor block. The combination of low-dose intrathecal bupivacaine (2.5 mg) and fentanyl (15–25 g) provides the desired analgesia by synergism. Although an epidural can be used, the disadvantages are that analgesia can be delayed and quite high doses may be required initially to prevent the mother bearing down in an involuntary way. It would, therefore, be anticipated that the mother would have a degree of motor impairment.

Further analgesia in this case was provided by intermittent 10 ml boluses of 0.1% bupivacaine with 0.0002% fentanyl. Dilutions of bupivacaine up to 0.0625% are found to be effective in providing analgesia with motor sparing when used with fentanyl.

Intermittent top-ups were administered by trained personnel to maintain analgesia in this patient. Top-ups were guided by breakthrough discomfort and by giving analgesia in this way, the amount of local anaesthetic is tailored to the individual patient's requirements. Patient-controlled epidural analgesia or intermittent boluses given by midwife or anaesthetist have a dose-sparing effect compared to a continuous epidural infusion, which is ideal in these circumstances.

Analgesia in the second stage of labour

Management of the second stage vaginal breech delivery relies on watchful expectancy to allow spontaneous delivery of the breech up to the umbilicus. Care should be taken to ensure that the cervix is fully dilated and the breech has descended to the pelvic floor before initiating active pushing. Delivery of the limbs, shoulders and the head is better assisted to decrease the morbidity to the baby from the birth. In this case, the plan was for an assisted breech delivery. Assisted delivery of the limbs, shoulders and the after-coming head requires good analgesia and some pelvic floor relaxation.

Analgesia must be extended into the second stage of labour. In this case, an epidural top-up of 15 ml of 0.1% bupivacaine and 0.0002% fentanyl was given on the diagnosis of full cervical dilatation to allow descent of the presenting part to the perineum before active pushing commenced. The mother did not require any further top-ups because she was comfortable with good perineal analgesia, but this must be carefully assessed and further top-ups must be given, if required, after active pushing has commenced.

Caesarean section

The possibility of an emergency Caesarean section should be anticipated, particularly in a breech presentation. The concerns and precautions are similar as for any Caesarean section. Anaesthesia may be required rapidly, so the anaesthetist must ensure that the mother's epidural is working well and that a good block for Caesarean section can be achieved by an epidural top-up of 20 ml of 0.5% bupivacaine with fentanyl. One disadvantage of the CSE technique is the delayed testing of the epidural catheter, although there is evidence that a catheter placed in the epidural space after a needle-through-needle CSE usually works well because the technique confirms correct identification of the epidural space.

If the mother needs a Caesarean section and does not have a working epidural *in situ*, then either a CSE or single-shot spinal anaesthetic is acceptable. Intra-operative events are similar to normal Caesarean sections, although the delivery of the after-coming head may be difficult and prolonged, and occasionally requires that a tocolytic be given. In preterm breech, the cervical segment may be inadequate leading to a classical uterine incision, which may cause more bleeding and impaired uterine contraction.

KEY LEARNING POINTS

1. Although vaginal delivery of a breech baby is becoming less common, it will never be possible to prevent all breech deliveries either because of maternal wish or late presentation of an uncomplicated breech labour.

2. The anaesthetic aims are as follows:
    a. To rapidly provide an epidural if the mother wishes it.
    b. Prevent premature maternal bearing down on an incompletely dilated cervix by ensuring good sacral analgesia.
    c. To use the lowest possible dose of local anaesthetic in an epidural or CSE to maximise maternal pushing in the second stage of labour.
    d. Provide good second stage analgesia to assist the delivery of the baby's shoulders and head.
    e. Have a tested and working epidural, so it can be used rapidly to establish anaesthesia if a Caesarean becomes necessary.

Further reading

Albrechtsen S, Rasmussen S, Irgens LM. Secular trends in perinatal and neonatal mortality in breech. *Acta Obstetrica et Gynaecologica Scandinavica* 2000; **79**: 508–12.

Collis RE, Davies DW, Aveling W. Randomised comparison of CSE and standard epidural analgesia in labour. *Lancet* 1995; **345**: 1413–16.

Croughan-Minihene MS, Pettiti DB, Gordis L, Golditch I. Morbidity among breech infants according to method of delivery. *Obstetrics and Gynaecology* 1990; **75**: 821–5.

Ferrante FM, Barber MJ, Segal M, Hughes NJ, Datta S. 0.0625% bupivacaine with 0.0002% fentanyl via PCEA for pain of labour and delivery. *Clinical Journal of Pain* 1995; **11**: 121–6.

Fung BK. Continuous epidural analgesia for painless labour does not increase the incidence of caesarean delivery. *Acta Anaesthesiologica Scandinavica* 2000; **38**: 79–84.

Gimovsky ML, Wallace RL, Schifrin BS, Paul RH. Randomised management of the non frank breech presentation at term: a preliminary report. *American Journal of Obstetrics and Gynecology* 1983; **146**: 34–40.

Hannah ME, Hannah WJ, Hewson SA, Hodnett ED, Saigal S, Willan AR. Planned caesarean section versus planned vaginal birth for breech presentation at term: a randomised multicentre trial. Term Breech Trial Collaborative Group. *Lancet* 2000; **356**: 1375–83.

Hepner DL, Gaiser RR, Cheek TG, Gutsche BB. Comparison of CSE and low dose epidural for labour analgesia. *Canadian Journal of Anaesthesia* 2000; **47**: 232–6.

Hickok DE, Gordon DC, Milberg JA, Williams MA, Daling JR. The frequency of breech presentation by gestational age at birth: a large population based study. *American Journal of Obstetrics and Gynecology* 1992; **166**: 851–2.

Hofmeyr GJ. External cephalic version for breech before term (Review). *Cochrane Database of Systematic Reviews* (Computer file) 2000; **2**: CD000084.

Hofmeyr GJ, Hannah ME. Planned caesarean section for term breech delivery (Review). *Cochrane Database of Systematic Reviews* (Computer file) 2000; **2**: CD000166.

Lucas DN, Ciccone GK, Yentis SM. Extending low dose epidural analgesia for emergency Caesarean section. A comparison of three solutions. *Anaesthesia* 1999; **54**: 1173–7.

Makris N, Xygakis A, Chinos A, Sakellaropoulos G, Michalas S. The management of breech presentation in the last three decades. *Clinical and Experimental Obstetrics and Gynecology* 1999; **26**: 178–80.

Oloffson C, Ekbolm A, Ekman-Ordebrg G, Irestedt L. Obstetric outcome following epidural analgesia with bupivacaine–adrenaline 0.25% or bupivacaine 0.125% with sufentanil: a prospective randomised control study in 1000 parturients. *Acta Anaesthesiologica Scandinavica* 1998; **42**: 284–92.

Palmer CM, Van Maren G, Nogami WM, Alves D. Bupivacaine augments intrathecal fentanyl for labor analgesia. *Anesthesiology* 1999; **91**: 84–9.

Sia AT, Chang JL. Epidural 0.2% ropivacaine for labour analgesia: patient controlled or continuous infusion? *Anaesthesia and Intensive Care* 1999; **27**: 154–8.

4

'CRASH' CAESAREAN SECTION

P.S. Sudheer and M. Stacey

CASE HISTORY

A 20-year-old lady was admitted to the labour ward with spontaneous rupture of her membranes. She was 38 weeks gestation and not in active labour. On vaginal examination, she had a pulsatile, prolapsed cord. An obstetric decision was made to deliver the foetus without further delay. The anaesthetist was informed that the baby had to be delivered immediately. A quick review of her notes revealed that she was fit and healthy, taking only iron tablets and had no allergies. The obstetricians had positioned her in the knee-to-chest position and the midwife was pushing the presenting part away from the cord.

A large intravenous cannula was sited and the opportunity was taken for a brief essential history from the patient focussing on past and present medical problems, history of medications and allergies, previous anaesthetic history and the booking weight. There was no indication of a difficult airway and there were no false, capped or crowned teeth. Verbal consent for postoperative diclofenac suppository was also obtained.

In the anaesthetic room, after full monitoring was established, she was turned onto her back and positioned with a left lateral tilt to establish left uterine displacement. The table was tilted head down. All this time, the midwife supported the presenting part well away from the cord. The patient was given 30 ml of 0.3 M sodium citrate orally.

Pre-oxygenation with four vital capacity breaths was performed and anaesthesia induced with thiopental 350 mg and suxamethonium 100 mg. Cricoid pressure was applied on loss of consciousness and her trachea was intubated in the presence of the scrubbed surgeon and assistant. She had a grade II laryngoscopic view and anaesthesia was maintained with oxygen, nitrous oxide and 1 MAC of isoflurane. Her lungs were ventilated to achieve an end-tidal carbon dioxide tension of 4.5 kPa. A healthy baby boy was delivered with Apgar scores of 9 and 10 at 1 and 5 min, respectively. Intravenous morphine 10 mg was injected following delivery. An orogastric tube was passed to empty her stomach contents and then removed. She was extubated awake and on her side. For postoperative analgesia, she was given regular paracetamol 1 g 6 hourly, rectal diclofenac sodium 100 mg followed by 50 mg 8 hourly and patient-controlled analgesia (PCA) morphine 1 mg bolus with a lockout of 5 min.

DEFINITION OF THE PROBLEM

Anaesthesia for Caesarean section has undergone a major change over the last decade with a swing away from general towards regional anaesthesia. However, certain indications warrant general anaesthesia and often occur in the middle of the night. Such indications include an obstetric emergency where there is insufficient time to establish a regional anaesthetic; a contraindication to a regional anaesthetic; or a patient's refusal to have a regional anaesthetic. The most stressful situation is where there is extreme urgency for Caesarean delivery requiring rapid establishment of general anaesthesia.

PATHOPHYSIOLOGY

Mendelson, in 1946, described the problems of gastric aspiration during obstetric anaesthesia. Inhalation of even small amounts of gastric secretions of low pH (often quoted as <2.5) can cause rapid onset of pulmonary oedema and respiratory distress known as Mendelson's syndrome. The obstetric patient is at risk of gastric regurgitation and aspiration during general anaesthesia because of reduced lower oesophageal sphincter tone and increased intra-gastric pressure as a result of compression from the gravid uterus.

In the supine position, the pregnant uterus compresses the vena cava and aorta, which can be demonstrated by radiological studies. Although obstruction of the aorta may not produce maternal symptoms, it can affect placental circulation and cause foetal asphyxia. Obstruction of the inferior vena cava, however, produces maternal symptoms, such as faintness, nausea, vomiting, pallor and sweating. These symptoms are the result of maternal hypotension and are described as the 'supine hypotension syndrome'. Hypotension results from a decrease in venous return and, therefore, a decrease in cardiac output. It is worsened by the onset of general anaesthesia, which causes further decreases in cardiac output.

The incidence of failed intubation during general anaesthesia for Caesarean section is greater than that in non-pregnant women. There are probably a number of factors independently contributing to this. These include: alterations in airway anatomy with pregnancy, the presence of enlarged breasts inhibiting the insertion of the laryngoscope, incorrectly applied cricoid pressure distorting laryngeal anatomy, the inexperience and greater anxiety of the anaesthetist aware of the risks to mother and baby of failed intubation and acid aspiration.

MANAGEMENT OPTIONS AND DISCUSSION

The term 'crash induction' was first used in 1957. Although initially there was no formal description of what a rapid sequence induction (RSI) entails regarding timing of drug administration and achieving a definitive airway, most anaesthetists now agree that the major components of RSI include:

- pre-oxygenation,

- prevention of aspiration pneumonitis,

- prevention of supine hypotension,

- preparation for a failed intubation.

Maternal morbidity and mortality has declined over the years partly because of widespread use of regional anaesthesia, as well as improvements in training, consultant supervision and the experience of obstetric anaesthetic trainees. There has also been greater understanding as well as preparedness among the anaesthetists.

Prolapse of the umbilical cord

Umbilical cord presentation is the presence of a segment of umbilical cord at the cervical os as the presenting part. Prolapse is present when the membrane has ruptured and the segment may be at any level from the upper vagina to outside the introitus. The only characteristic sign is the finding of a palpable or visible cord in the vagina. It then requires an assessment of the foetal condition. Cord accident (presentation or prolapse) is an indication for immediate Caesarean section if the baby is alive and vaginal delivery cannot be effected immediately.

Once the patient presents with a cord prolapse, it is essential to reassure the mother, establish venous access and obtain blood for a full blood count, blood group and save, and electrolytes. The mother should be positioned in a knee-to-chest position or an exaggerated Sim's position (semi-prone with the bottom half of the body extended and the upper flexed at the hip and knees) to minimise cord compression. It is not possible to induce safe anaesthesia in either of these positions, and the mother will have to be turned onto her back and kept slightly head down. It is also required to keep the pressure off the cord, and where necessary, replace the cord in the vagina to keep it warm and prevent vasospasm (fundic reduction). A urinary catheter should be passed and the bladder filled with 500–700 ml of normal saline. This manoeuvre elevates the presenting part and maintains foetal condition while preparation for Caesarean section is made.

Preparation for emergency general anaesthesia

At the start of each shift, the resident obstetric anaesthetist should check the anaesthetic equipment and anaesthetic machine according to the Association of Anaesthetists of Great Britain and Ireland guidelines. The anaesthetist should also ensure that drugs for an emergency Caesarean section are readily available, and it is common practice to draw up thiopental and suxamethonium fresh every day and keep them refrigerated. The difficult airway trolley should be checked and should contain an array of different sizes of laryngoscopes: McCoy, Polio and short-handled laryngoscopes. It is essential to have a bougie available. The laryngeal mask airway is becoming more commonly used in the difficult airway scenario, even in obstetrics. Facilities to provide a surgical airway should be available and it is important that the resident is well versed with a safe 'failed intubation drill' (see Figure 4.1) and is familiar with the equipments in the trolley. It is advisable for trainees starting in obstetric anaesthesia to practise a difficult airway scenario and the local failed intubation drill on training lists with consultants.

Prior to induction of anaesthesia, the patient is pre-oxygenated and the conventional method of pre-oxygenation consists of breathing 100% oxygen for 3–5 min. This denitrogenates the patient's lungs and effectively provides an oxygen reserve of around 2 l in the functional residual capacity of the lung. Bernard *et al.* described effective pre-oxygenation after four vital capacity breathes, even in pregnant women. It is best not to ventilate the patient prior to intubation to avoid gastric insufflation, thereby increasing the risk of regurgitation. High-volume suction should be ready if required. Anaesthesia should preferably be induced with the patient on an operating table in theatre with the surgeon and assistant scrubbed and ready to proceed immediately after induction of anaesthesia and securing the airway.

Protection from gastric aspiration

To reduce the danger of aspiration, it is a common practice to reduce the quantity of gastric secretions as well as reduce the acidity of stomach contents. Reduction of gastric volume and pH is usually achieved by a combination of a histamine (H_2) receptor antagonist (e.g. ranitidine) or a proton pump inhibitor (e.g. omeprazole) and oral sodium citrate.

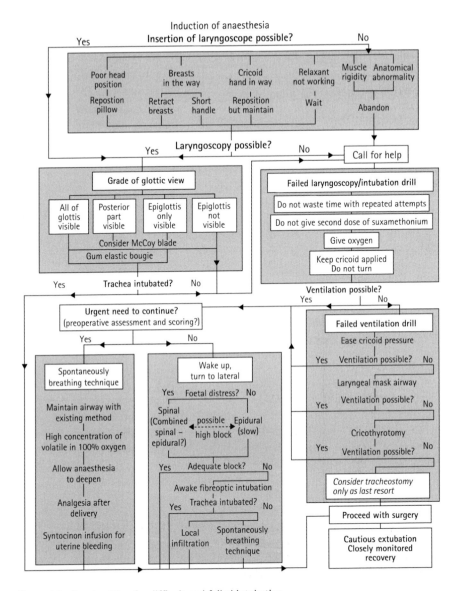

Figure 4.1 – An algorithm for difficult and failed intubation.

In 1961, Sellick described cricoid pressure as a technique to prevent regurgitation of stomach contents during induction of anaesthesia. The technique and the timing of application of the cricoid pressure vary among different practitioners and appear to be more commonly practised in the UK. Inappropriately applied cricoid pressure can contribute to difficult laryngoscopy, and Hartsilver and Vanner demonstrated that cricoid pressure applied with a force of 44 N (equivalent to a weight of 4.4 kg), especially when pressure was applied backwards and upwards, was more likely to produce airway obstruction. They showed that a pressure of 30 N applied in a backward direction would not obstruct the airway and is sufficient to prevent regurgitation of gastric contents. (In practical terms, 10 N is the force required to register 1 kg when applied to a weighing scale.) The extubation period is as crucial as the induction. The stomach should be emptied intraoperatively with a large orogastric tube and the patient's trachea extubated only when awake.

Aortocaval compression

Various methods are described to relieve aortocaval compression including a left lateral tilt of 15–20°, using a Cardiff wedge or even a full lateral position. Bamber measured the cardiac output in left and right lateral positions and found that the cardiac output was significantly reduced in the right tilt positions, while there was no significant reduction in cardiac output with different degrees of left lateral tilt.

Induction of anaesthesia

Conventionally, thiopental and suxamethonium have been used for induction of anaesthesia. A pre-calculated dose of thiopental (5 mg/kg) is given followed soon after by suxamethonium (1.5 mg/kg) for its rapid onset and its quick offset, which is an advantage if intubation is unsuccessful. However, some would argue that a waning suxamethonium level causes a greater risk of aspiration and a more difficult intubation than using a longer acting non-depolarising neuromuscular-blocking agent. It is also worthwhile mentioning that there is a tendency among inexperienced anaesthetists in the heat of the situation to attempt intubation prior to the establishment of muscle relaxation.

There are variations in practice with regard to the timing of suxamethonium administration. Some anaesthetists give it immediately following thiopental, while others delay administration until the patient loses consciousness. A range of induction agents has been used, such as ketamine, etomidate, propofol and inhalation induction. High-dose vecuronium and rocuronium have been used instead of suxamethonium.

Analgesia for the procedure is achieved with opiates, though administration is delayed until after delivery because of the fear of neonatal respiratory depression. Fentanyl or alfentanil are sometimes injected during induction to reduce the stress response to laryngoscopy in pre-eclamptic women. Boluses of remifentanil in doses greater than 1 mcg/kg obtund the stress response, but doses greater than 1.5 mcg/kg can cause hypotension.

KEY LEARNING POINTS

1. Maternal mortality and morbidity have declined dramatically over the years partly due to the importance given to the practice of regional anaesthesia.

2. There have been significant improvements in communication among the medical team as well as training and senior cover of labour wards.

3. The role of general anaesthesia for Caesarean section will continue to decline with the danger that the resident anaesthetist in obstetric units may not have the skills or experience to conduct a safe obstetric anaesthetic in an emergency.

4. As with all emergency anaesthesia, a relevant pre-operative evaluation should be made with particular emphasis on the airway, and measures to reduce the risk of aspiration instituted.

5. Consider urgency for delivery. If the obstetricians advise immediate delivery, then general anaesthesia may be the preferred option.

6. However, in experienced hands, spinal anaesthesia may still be quicker.

7. Adequate experience and assistance is required.

8. Pre-oxygenation, left uterine displacement and monitoring are mandatory.

9. Having taken the decision for immediate delivery, the surgeons must be scrubbed and ready to proceed soon after induction.

10. Avoid hyperventilation during maintenance of anaesthesia to avoid foetal alkalosis.

11. Provide adequate postoperative analgesia with a combination of simple analgesics and opiates.

12. Empty stomach with a wide orogastric tube and extubate awake.

Further reading

Bamber J. Aortocaval compression: the effect of changing the amount and direction of lateral tilt on maternal cardiodynamics. *International Journal of Obstetric Anesthesia* 2000; **9**: 167.

Bienarz I, Crothogini JJ, Curachet E. Aortocaval compression by uterus in late human pregnancy. *American Journal of Obstetrics and Gynecology* 1968; **100**: 203–17.

Hartsilver EL, Vanner RG, Bewley J, Clayton T. Gastric pressure during emergency caesarian section under general anaesthesia. *British Journal of Anaesthesia* 1999; **82**: 752–4.

Hartsilver EL, Vanner RG. Airway obstruction with cricoid pressure. *Anaesthesia* 2000; **55**: 600.

Howard BK, Goodson JH, Mengert WF. Supine hypotension in late pregnancy. *Obstetric and Gynaecology* 1953; **1**: 371–7.

Kerr MG, Scott DB, Samuel E. Studies of the inferior vena cava in late pregnancy. *British Medical Journal* 1964; **1**: 532–3.

Mendelson CL. The aspiration of stomach contents into the lungs during obstetric anaesthesia. *American Journal of Obstetric and Gynecology* 1946; **52**: 191–205.

Morris S. Management of difficult and failed intubation in obstetrics. *British Journal of Anaesthesia, CEPD Reviews* 2001; **1**: 118.

O'Hare, Mc Atamney D, Mirakhur RK, Hughes D, Carabine V. Bolus of remifentanil for control of haemodynamic response to tracheal intubation during rapid sequence induction. *British Journal of Anaesthesia* 1999; **82**: 283–5.

Sellick BA. Cricoid pressure to control regurgitation of stomach contents during induction of anaesthesia. *Lancet* 1961; **2**: 404–6.

Stept WJ, Safar P. Rapid induction/intubation for prevention of gastric content aspiration. *Anesthesia and Analgesia* 1970; **49**: 633–6.

Thwaites AJ, Rice CP, Smith I. A questionnaire survey of routine conduct and continued management during a failed intubation. *Anaesthesia* 1999; **54**: 376–81.

5

DIABETES IN PREGNANCY

J. Curtis and C. Farley

CASE HISTORY

A pregnant, 34-year-old insulin dependent diabetic underwent several surgical procedures in the mid-trimester, culminating in an elective Caesarean section at 28 weeks gestation.

Her diabetes was diagnosed at the age of 18 years. Prior to pregnancy, her diabetic control was poor with persistently elevated levels of glycosylated haemoglobin (HbA1c) and repeated hospital admissions for diabetic ketoacidosis (DKA). Her diabetes was complicated by

- nephropathy and hypertension;

- retinopathy;

- peripheral neuropathy with foot ulceration and bilateral neuropathic ankle joints;

- severe autonomic neuropathy with postural hypotension, gastroparesis, vomiting, persistent diarrhoea and lack of awareness of the symptoms of hypoglycaemia;

- obesity with a pre-pregnancy body mass index of $42.5 \, \text{kg/m}^2$.

On becoming pregnant, she remained under the care of her diabetic physician, a nephrologist and an obstetrician with a special interest in diabetes. Enalapril, which is teratogenic, was changed to methyldopa to control her hypertension. Elevated plasma concentrations of urea and creatinine were noted.

She spent much of her early pregnancy in hospital because of profound vomiting. Poor diabetic control led to episodes of hypoglycaemia, and the associated dehydration superimposed a degree of pre-renal failure on her existing nephropathy. This was treated with intravenous fluids, sliding scale insulin, domperidone and metoclopramide. By 14 weeks gestation, urine protein loss was greater than 10 g/day, which in association with poor nutritional intake, led to marked hypoproteinaemia. A nasojejunostomy tube was placed and enteral feeding commenced. At 16 weeks gestation, she developed a popliteal vein thrombosis, which was treated with subcutaneous low molecular weight heparin. After a short spell at home, she was re-admitted at 23 weeks gestation with a swollen, painful right thigh, suggesting an extension of the popliteal vein thrombosis. Intravenous heparin was instituted, the swelling became more painful and there was a fall in haemoglobin concentration. An urgent MRI scan confirmed the presence of a large haematoma in the right vastus lateralis muscle, so heparin was discontinued. She was transfused 4 units of red blood cells and 2 units of fresh frozen plasma and scheduled for fasciotomy and drainage.

On examination, she was pyrexial (37.9°C), pulse was 100 beats/min and blood pressure 160/95 mmHg. She had a patchy sensory loss to fine touch in her lower limbs and there was loss of the Valsalva response. Her ECG was normal and blood results are summarised in Table 5.1. Her medication included intravenous sliding scale insulin and dextrose, methyldopa, domperidone and metoclopramide. All forms of heparin were discontinued before surgery.

She was premedicated with intravenous ranitidine 50 mg, followed by oral sodium citrate 30 ml. A second intravenous line and a right radial arterial line were inserted before induction of anaesthesia. A rapid sequence induction with cricoid pressure was performed with left lateral tilt position after pre-oxygenation for 5 min. In addition to thiopental (375 mg) and suxamethonium (100 mg), alfentanil (1 mg) was given to obtund the hypertensive response to laryngoscopy and intubation. Anaesthesia was maintained with isoflurane in 50% nitrous oxide in oxygen. Muscle relaxation was maintained with atracurium (40 mg) and morphine (5 mg) given for analgesia. Routine monitoring was used with the addition of direct arterial blood pressure measurement.

The affected muscle looked ischaemic, the dead tissue was excised and a large haematoma was evacuated from the thigh with partial wound closure. Following reversal of residual neuromuscular blockade, the trachea was extubated with the patient awake in the full left lateral position. She was transferred to the high dependency unit (HDU) for close postoperative observation and monitoring. Sliding scale insulin was continued and patient-controlled analgesia (PCA) morphine was started.

Surgery was required on four subsequent occasions for cleaning and debridement of the infected wound and wound closure. A Hickmann line was inserted as venous access had become extremely difficult. A further 6 units of blood were transfused over this 4-week period. Anaesthesia for these procedures was exactly as described above. The patient adamantly refused regional anaesthesia at all times.

By 26 weeks gestation, there was reverse flow in the umbilical arteries on Doppler study and gross intrauterine growth retardation (IUGR); therefore, elective Caesarean section was scheduled at 28 weeks gestation. The patient was by this time re-established on low molecular weight heparin, dexamethasone was given to improve foetal lung maturation and sliding scale insulin with dextrose was controlling her diabetes. There was a deterioration in renal function with an increase in urea to 19.7 mmol/l and creatinine to 320 µmol/l, though urine output remained satisfactory. She was treated with labetolol for her persistently elevated blood pressure, and her blood glucose level remained labile.

Anaesthesia for Caesarean section was the same as for her previous surgery except that syntocinon (5 units) and morphine (10 mg) were given after clamping the umbilical cord. A 900 g live female infant was delivered, its trachea intubated and it was taken to the neonatal intensive care unit. The baby was subsequently diagnosed with a complex cardiac abnormality and died on the neonatal unit aged 4 months.

Postoperatively, the patient was again nursed on HDU where she developed a paralytic ileus. Her renal function deteriorated, she became oliguric and was transferred to the regional renal unit for dialysis. Approximately 1 year later, the patient died from complications of renal failure.

Table 5.1 – Pre-operative blood results.

Haematology	
Haemoglobin	9.9 g/dl
White blood count	$2.5 \times 10^9/l$
Platelet count	$212 \times 10^9/l$
Biochemistry	
Na	136 mmol/l
K	4.7 mmol/l
Urea	17.5 mmol/l
Creatinine	284 µmol/l
Glucose	7 mmol/l
Albumen	16 g/dl
Coagulation	
KCCT	
Patient	45 s
Control	30 s

Table 5.2 – Classification of diabetes in pregnancy.

Class	Age of onset	Duration of diabetes (years)	Description
A$_1$	Any	Any	Gestational diabetes – no insulin
A$_2$	Any	Any	Gestational diabetes – insulin required
B	>20	<10	Insulin – no vascular complications
C	10–19	10–19	Insulin – no vascular complications
D	<10	>20	Insulin – moderate vascular disease, e.g. hypertension, retinitis and transitory albuminuria
*F, R, T and H	Any	Any	All insulin dependent diabetics with F *nephropathy*, R *proliferative retinopathy*, T *renal transplant* and H *ischaemic heart disease*

*Categories F, R, T and H are associated with poor foetal outcome and a significant increase in maternal morbidity and in the case of category H, mortality.

DEFINITION OF THE PROBLEM

Diabetes mellitus is the most common medical disorder complicating pregnancy. Babies of diabetic mothers are at significant risk of stillbirth and congenital abnormality, macrosomia and neonatal hypoglycaemia. While there is usually a favourable outcome in the well controlled, uncomplicated parturient, poor diabetic control and diabetes-related complications influence maternal and foetal outcome. In addition, complex diabetic patients may require repeated surgery and anaesthesia in the antenatal period, which poses a further risk. These factors combine to make the complex pregnant diabetic a challenge to manage successfully.

In 1949, Priscilla White produced a classification of diabetes in pregnancy (Table 5.2). Although this classification is outdated as it was developed at a time when the associated foetal mortality was high, it allows clinicians to focus on those factors that pose most risk to mother and infant.

PATHOPHYSIOLOGY

Glucose homeostasis is altered in pregnancy and may predispose the diabetic parturient to episodes of hypo- and hyperglycaemia. In early pregnancy, increases in oestrogen and progesterone lead to beta-cell hyperplasia and increased insulin secretion. While increased peripheral utilisation of glucose causes lower maternal fasting glucose levels. Glycogen deposition increases in peripheral tissues, accompanied by a decrease in hepatic glucose production. Therefore, diabetics commonly experience periods of hypoglycaemia. Conversely, later in pregnancy, there is postreceptor resistance to insulin. The presumed mechanism involves increases in the counter regulatory hormones, placental lactogen, placental growth hormone, cortisol and progesterone resulting in increased insulin requirements of approximately 30% above pre-pregnancy dosage.

Maternal consequences of diabetes

Factors predisposing to hypoglycaemia include emesis, tight glucose control and episodes of severe hypoglycaemia before pregnancy. Factors predisposing to hyperglycaemia with the potential for DKA include poor physician management, emesis, beta-adrenergic agonist therapy, infection, non-compliance with diabetic treatment and steroid therapy. Both profound hypoglycaemia and DKA are associated with severe foetal distress and poor outcome.

Some diabetic complications can progress in pregnancy and retinopathy may be accelerated. However, nephropathy is not usually worsened but is associated with an increased risk of pre-eclampsia, IUGR and foetal distress. In our case, dehydration secondary to vomiting, poor blood pressure control and finally, paralytic ileus with large fluid loss into the gut, caused renal deterioration. It is unclear whether pregnancy accelerates the progression of either somatic or autonomic neuropathy. Diabetes is associated with an increased risk of pregnancy-induced hypertension, polyhydramnios and Caesarean section.

Foetal complications of diabetes

Macrosomia is relatively common and is associated with shoulder dystocia and birth trauma.

Neonatal hypoglycaemia is presumably the result of sustained foetal hyperinsulinaemia, developed in response to chronic intrauterine hyperglycaemia and acute maternal hyperglycaemia. There is a higher incidence of neonatal respiratory distress syndrome and neonatal hyperbilirubinaemia in infants of diabetic mothers. There is an increased incidence of stillbirth and foetal distress leading to premature delivery. Foetal hypoxia may reflect reduced uteroplacental blood flow, which may be decreased by up to 45% in the third trimester. In addition, glycosylated haemoglobin is a poor carrier of oxygen and leads to impaired neonatal oxygen extraction.

With improved care in the diabetic parturient, congenital malformations have emerged as the leading cause of perinatal mortality. Abnormalities particularly affect the cardiovascular and central nervous system as well as urogenital and gastrointestinal systems. Hyperglycaemia in the first 7 weeks post-conception, the critical period of organogenesis, may cause foetal malformation. The incidence of congenital malformation is seven to 10 times higher than in non-diabetic mothers; however, with strict pre-conception glycaemic control this can be reduced.

MANAGEMENT OPTIONS AND DISCUSSION

Obstetric management

Obstetric care of the diabetic patient should be multidisciplinary with specific care commencing before conception. Awareness of the presence of complicating factors allows appropriate counselling. Close maternal–foetal surveillance allows the optimum timing and mode of delivery to be determined.

Whatever the mode of delivery, there must be strict glucose control to prevent rebound hypoglycaemia in the infant. In the labouring diabetic, insulin requirements are often small. Most obstetricians avoid a prolonged second stage as this increases foetal acidaemia. Elective Caesarean section should be scheduled early in the day to avoid prolonged fasting. Dextrose, potassium and insulin infusions should be given via a dedicated line and adjusted according to unit protocol, usually to maintain blood glucose between 4 and 9 mmol/l. A second intravenous line is sited to give crystalloid, colloid and blood products. There is usually a decrease in insulin requirements after delivery of the placenta with subsequent risk of hypoglycaemia. When normal diet is resumed in the post-partum phase, the usual daily insulin regimen can be restarted.

Our patient became pregnant when her diabetic control was poor despite counselling from her physician. The presence of renal failure, retinopathy and significant peripheral and autonomic neuropathy places her in category F on the White classification, a grade associated with poor outcome.

Substituting her enalapril with methyldopa doubtless compromised blood pressure control although resistant hypertension was probably more due to accelerating vascular disease in pregnancy and may have been a factor in her deteriorating renal function and poor placental function. The vomiting that occurred throughout pregnancy, but particularly in the first trimester, was probably a combination of hyperemesis gravidarum and her longstanding diabetic gastroparesis. Profuse vomiting led to a degree of pre-renal failure and hypoglycaemia and with the protein–losing nephropathy contributed to hypoproteinaemia. Enteral feeding via jejunostomy tube helped to improve nutrition. Similar successful management in gastroparesis has been described.

The combination of pregnancy and diabetes produces hypercoagulability, and the presence of dehydration and immobility due to joint problems further contributed to our patient's popliteal vein thrombosis. Muscle infarction, though rare, has been described in poorly controlled diabetics. The initial misdiagnosis and subsequent anticoagulation led to haematoma formation requiring surgical intervention.

Anaesthetic management

The optimal anaesthetic management of pregnant diabetics is based on studies of non-pregnant diabetics and pregnant non-diabetics. Unsurprisingly, the aims are to avoid hypotension and hypoxia, to minimise the disruption to oral intake, thus maintaining adequate glucose levels, to minimise the risk of gastric aspiration, and to monitor cerebral function by maintaining verbal contact whenever possible. Thus, regional anaesthesia is desirable. Spinal anaesthesia in diabetics has been associated with an increase in foetal acidosis, possibly due to maternal hypotension. However, when management includes volume expansion with non-dextrose containing solutions, aggressive treatment of hypotension to achieve systolic pressure above 100 mmHg and glucose levels are well controlled at the time of delivery, the incidence of foetal acidosis is the same as in non-diabetic patients. During labour, epidural analgesia minimises the stress response and can be used for instrumental or Caesarean delivery as required.

There is little evidence as to what is the best method of anaesthesia for non-obstetric procedures in pregnant diabetics. Avoidance of hypoxia, hypotension and gastric aspiration are important, and many authors suggest regional anaesthesia is preferable for mother and baby.

We were faced with a pregnant, diabetic, obese, anticoagulated, hypertensive lady with deteriorating renal function, and severe autonomic and peripheral neuropathy. Management decisions were limited by an absolute and consistent refusal of any form of regional anaesthesia. Initially, anticoagulation and pyrexia were clinical contraindications to a regional technique. The disadvantages of general anaesthesia were the added risk of aspiration in the presence of gastroparesis, hypertension at laryngoscopy and the increased risk of hypoxia in the obese. Due to deranged renal function and hypoproteinaemia, drug pharmacokinetics were unpredictable, a factor of concern particularly in the postoperative period when opioids were needed for analgesia. A 'stiff joint' syndrome has been described in diabetics resulting in limited movement at the atlanto-occipital joint and difficulty with laryngoscopy.

Usually, a regional technique is preferable for Caesarean section, although severe autonomic neuropathy leading to profound hypotension is a major concern. Epidural anaesthesia or a combined epidural with low dose spinal allows a more gradual onset of anaesthesia, thus preventing profound precipitous falls in blood pressure. Epidural analgesia could then be used in the postoperative period.

Opiates cause a decrease in gut motility and together with autonomic gut paresis may have contributed to our patient's postoperative paralytic ileus.

KEY LEARNING POINTS

1. Diabetes mellitus is the most common medical condition affecting pregnancy.

2. The presence of diabetic complications adversely affects foetal and maternal outcome.

3. There is a relatively high incidence of perinatal mortality in diabetics in the UK.

4. A multidisciplinary approach to care should begin before conception with scrupulous glucose control, close foetal surveillance and optimum timing of delivery.

5. Where possible, regional analgesia and anaesthesia should be employed for delivery.

6. Whatever technique is selected, hypotension and hypoxia must be avoided and normoglycaemia maintained.

Further reading

Carr ME. Diabetes mellitus: a hypercoaguable state. *Journal of Diabetes and its Complications* 2001; **15**: 44–54.

Casson IF, Clarke CA, Howard CV, *et al.* Outcomes of pregnancy in insulin dependent diabetic women: results of a five year population cohort study. *British Medical Journal* 1997; **315**: 275–8.

Combs CA, Kitzmiller JL. Diabetic nephropathy and pregnancy. *Clinical Obstetrics and Gynecology* 1991; **34**: 505–15.

Datta S, Brown WU. Acid–base status in diabetic mothers and their infants following general or spinal anaesthesia for caesarean section. *Anesthesiology* 1977; **47**: 272–6.

Datta S, Kitzmiller JL, Naulty, *et al.* Acid base status of diabetic mothers and their infants following spinal anesthesia for caesarean section. *Anesthesia and Analgesia* 1982; **61**: 662–5.

Davies MJ, Rathbone BJ, McNally PG, Youde JH, Goddard WP. Management of severe gastroparesis diabeticorum. *British Medical Journal* 1995; **310**:1331–2.

Diabetes Control and Complications Trial Research Group. Pregnancy outcomes in the diabetes control and complications trial. *American Journal of Obstetrics and Gynecology* 1996; **174**: 1343–53.

Dowling CJ, Kumar S, Boulton AJM. A difficult case: severe gastroparesis diabeticorum in a young patient with insulin dependent diabetes. *British Medical Journal* 1995; **310**: 308–9.

Grogoriadis E, Fam AG, Starok M, Ang LC. Skeletal muscle infarction in diabetes mellitus. *Journal of Rheumatology* 2000; **227**: 1063–8.

Hawthorne G, Robson S, Ryall EA, *et al*. Prospective population based survey of diabetic pregnancy outcome: results of the northern diabetic pregnancy audit. *British Medical Journal* 1994; **315**: 79–81.

Jacober SJ, Narayan A, Strodel WE, Vinik AI. Jejunostomy feeding in the management of gastroparesis diabeticorum. *Diabetes Care* 1986; **9**: 217–19.

Klein BEK, Moss SE, Klein R. Effect of pregnancy on the progression of diabetic retinopathy. *Diabetes Care* 1990; **13**: 34.

Madsen H, Ditzel J. Changes in red cell oxygen transport in diabetic pregnancy. *American Journal of Obstetrics and Gynecology* 1982; **143**: 421.

McBeth C, Murrin K. Subarachnoid block for a case of multiple system atrophy. *Anaesthesia* 1997; **52**: 884–5.

Nylund L, Lunnell NO, Lewander R, *et al*. Uteroplacental blood flow in diabetic pregnancy; measurements with indium-113m and a computer linked gamma camera. *American Journal of Obstetrics and Gynecology* 1976; **144**: 298.

Robert MF, Neff RK, Hubbell JP, *et al*. Association between maternal diabetes and the respiratory – distress syndrome in the newborn. *New England Journal of Medicine* 1976; **294**: 357–60.

Salzarulo HH, Taylor LA. Diabetic 'stiff joint syndrome' as a cause of difficult endotracheal intubation. *Anesthesiology* 1986; **64**: 366–8.

Watkins PJ, Thomas PK. Diabetes mellitus and the nervous system. *Journal of Neurology and Neurosurgery and Psychiatry* 1998; **65**: 620–32.

White P. Pregnancy complicating diabetes. *American Journal of Medicine* 1949; **7**: 609–16.

Yen SSC. Endocrine regulation of metabolic homeostasis during pregnancy. *Clinical Obstetrics and Gynecology* 1973; **16**: 130.

6

DRUG ABUSE IN PREGNANCY

S. Lloyd Jones and J. Griffiths

CASE HISTORY

A 28-year-old primiparous woman, who had a history of heroin abuse and known to be HIV positive, presented to the delivery suite at midnight in advanced labour. She had booked late in her pregnancy at 26 weeks gestation and had been enrolled in the local drug service clinic at this time. She was keen to reduce her drug intake during pregnancy and delivery. She was converted to oral methadone and stabilised on a dose of 20 mg a day by the drug rehabilitation clinic. Her hepatitis screen was negative but she refused further investigation into her CD4 count; so in view of her positive HIV status, plans were made for an elective Caesarean section with antiviral cover at 39 weeks gestation. She was otherwise well and denied the use of other illicit drugs.

At 38 weeks gestation, she presented to the delivery suite in established labour requesting analgesia. Initial examination found the cervix to be 6 cm dilated with prolonged Type II decelerations on the cardiotocograph (CTG). The obstetrician felt an urgent Caesarean section was indicated. Venous access was secured in the lateral aspect of the foot, after several fruitless attempts to cannulate an upper limb vein.

During the assessment period, the woman and her partner were aggressive and uncooperative, and it was felt by the anaesthetist that a general anaesthetic would be more appropriate. As the partner would not be able to attend the delivery, he became more aggressive and threatened the medical staff with physical violence. The mother then pulled out her cannula, and left the labour room, bleeding onto the delivery suite floor. Senior members of staff felt that the partner was aggravating the situation, so the hospital security was called. After the partner was removed by the security officer, the mother was more cooperative and allowed anaesthesia to proceed.

Recannulation was achieved with an intravenous line in the external jugular vein and general anaesthesia proceeded uneventfully. After antacid prophylaxis was given, a standard rapid sequence induction of thiopental 400 mg and succinyl choline 100 mg was carried out. Anaesthesia was maintained with oxygen/nitrous oxide/isoflurane with muscle relaxation provided by atracurium 30 mg. At appropriate times during the procedure, syntocinon 10 IU, co-amoxiclav 1.2 g, fentanyl 100 µg, and morphine 10 mg were given. Reversal of the neuromuscular blockade was achieved with neostigmine 2.5 mg and glycopyrronium 0.5 mg.

The baby had Apgar scores of 4 at 1 min and 8 at 5 min, and was admitted to the neonatal unit for observation. He subsequently showed some mild signs of withdrawal, which did not require any drug treatment. Formula feeding was established to reduce the risk of vertical transmission of HIV infection.

The patient made a good postoperative recovery. Patient-controlled anaesthesia (PCA) morphine was set initially to deliver a 1 mg bolus with a 5-min lockout, but it was evident that this was not providing sufficient analgesia. The bolus was gradually increased to 3 mg before satisfactory analgesia was obtained. Regular paracetemol and diclofenac were also prescribed and the PCA was removed on the 2nd postoperative day. The usual dose of oral methadone was given throughout the hospital stay and she was discharged home on the 5th postoperative day with appropriate social support.

DESCRIPTION OF THE PROBLEM

Illicit drug use during pregnancy is widespread. Most studies on prevalence come from the USA, where it is estimated that between 7.5% and 20% of women take illicit drugs during pregnancy.

1. Substance abuse during pregnancy is associated with poor physical and mental health in the mother.

2. An increased perinatal morbidity and mortality.

3. Associated factors, such as infection with blood-borne viruses, also adversely affect the health of mother and baby.

PATHOPHYSIOLOGY

General problems

It is well documented that drug abusers may have many medical problems resulting either directly from the drug abuse or from the lifestyle of the abuser (poor nutrition, cigarette smoking and homelessness); these have implications in pregnancy. Overdose may be fatal. On the other hand, withdrawal in pregnancy can cause miscarriage in the first trimester, foetal compromise and premature labour in later pregnancy.

Drug abuse affects all systems of the body (Table 6.1).

Cardiac problems include anaemia, endocarditis, arrhythmias, myocardial ischaemia and infarction.

Injecting drug users are 10 times more likely to acquire a chest infection than the general population. Pulmonary vascular granulomatosis may occur in users when crushed tablets intended for oral use are injected intravenously. Granuloma formation is an immune reaction to the talc that is used in the tablet to carry the active drug. The illness presents with progressive shortness of breath in association with a productive cough. Inhaling heroin fumes may cause histamine release and asthma.

Infective problems are common, ranging from local skin infections to human immunodeficiency virus (HIV) infection. Skin infections range in severity from abscesses and cellulitis, through thrombophlebitis to necrotising fascitis. Endocarditis, usually of the tricuspid valve, may result from locally infected sites. Septicaemia is caused by endocarditis in 40% of cases in intravenous drug users. The majority, however, occur as a result of soft tissue infection in the groin area around the femoral vein. Osteomyelitis and septic arthritis may occur by haematogenous spread from infected skin sites.

Recent case reports have highlighted *Clostridium novyi* and *Clostridium botulinum* as a cause of death and serious morbidity among injecting drug users. Abscesses at the

Table 6.1 – Effect of drug abuse on body systems.

Cardiac
  Anaemia
  Endocarditis
  Arrhythmias
  Myocardial ischaemia/infarction
Respiratory
  Chest infection
  Pulmonary vascular granulomatosis
Bacterial infection
  Skin abscess
  Cellulitis
  Thrombophlebitus
  Necrotising fascitis
Viral infection
  HIV
  Hepatitis B and C

site of injection produce a neurotoxin, which causes an acute symmetrical descending paralysis of cranial, peripheral and autonomic nerves.

Substance abuse in pregnancy is a significant risk factor for HIV. Recent investigation into the prevalence of HIV infection among pregnant women showed a prevalence of 1:520 in London and 1:5700 elsewhere in the UK. HIV infection is transmitted vertically from mother to unborn baby at a rate of 15–25%.

Drug–specific problems

Opioids

The opioids most commonly abused are diamorphine (heroin) and methadone. Heroin is the drug of choice for most addicts because it enters the central nervous system (CNS) rapidly because of its high lipid solubility, thus giving a quicker and more intense 'high' to the user.

Although the incidence of congenital malformations is not increased by the use of opioids alone before or during pregnancy, neonates regularly exposed to opioids during pregnancy are at risk of opioid withdrawal in utero and following birth. Signs of neonatal withdrawal syndrome include tremors, seizures, sneezing, fever, sweating, diarrhoea, vomiting and poor feeding. Signs are usually evident within 48 h of delivery but can take up to 2 weeks with methadone usage, due to its long half-life.

Given the chaotic lifestyle that usually accompanies heroin dependence and the risk to the foetus of acute withdrawal, the aim is to stabilise and then reduce drug intake. Many of the adverse effects of opioid abuse are due to the use of short-acting drugs, which cause fluctuating maternal levels. Methadone is the drug of choice for opioid substitution because it is legal, can be administered orally, and is of proven benefit and safety. It has a long duration of action and can be given as a once daily dose that provides relatively constant blood levels. However, it has actions and effects in common with the drugs it replaces, which increase as the dose increases. Substitution with methadone not only reduces polydrug use, but also offers the contact and opportunity for comprehensive medical care in a multidisciplinary setting.

It has been suggested that opioid detoxification should be carried out slowly if at all during pregnancy and restricted to the mid-trimester because of a theoretical risk of intrauterine death and/or early delivery. Others feel that the risk to the foetus is not a major problem (although acute foetal distress has been noted in the foetus on administering naloxone to the mother). Pregnant women using opioids should be offered detoxification with the objective of achieving the lowest dose compatible with reasonable maternal stability.

Studies of pregnant women receiving methadone have shown that plasma levels decrease during pregnancy because of an increased fluid space and a large tissue reservoir. There may also be altered metabolism by the placenta and foetus.

Pregnant woman may, therefore, genuinely require an increase in methadone. Similarly, in the postnatal period, a reversal of these effects may lead to increased methadone levels with potential toxic effects. Significant use of heroin is associated with an increased risk of preterm delivery, which is reduced by stabilisation on methadone. Women on methadone should continue to receive it in labour.

Cocaine

Cocaine is one of the major drug dependencies complicating pregnancy and it is a specifically well-recognised problem in the USA. In the UK, the level of awareness of this common problem needs to be improved.

The systemic effects of cocaine are caused by block of reuptake of noradrenaline and dopamine from synapses in the CNS and sympathetic nervous systems, thus, potentiating the effects of these neurotransmitters. The resulting high catecholamine levels cause vasoconstriction, tachycardia, hypertension and probably increased uterine contractility. Most pregnancy complications arise from this peripheral action. Chronic abuse causes tachyphylaxis resulting from depletion of presynaptic neurotransmitters.

'Crack' cocaine is heat stable and can be smoked and absorbed through alveolar membranes. It can also be 'snorted' in powder form or taken intravenously. Cocaine is metabolised by plasma and hepatic cholinesterases. The pharmacological effects may be exaggerated in pregnant women due to their reduced plasma cholinesterase activity. The metabolites are excreted in the urine within 48–72 h of use.

Cocaine has many adverse effects on pregnancy and the health of the foetus. There is a controversial link between cocaine use and the risk of congenital abnormalities. Intrauterine growth retardation is the most consistent finding in all studies. Preterm delivery, as with many forms of drug abuse, is more common. Labour may be precipitated by a large intravenous dose of cocaine, a method sometimes used by an addicted mother to induce her labour. Placental abruption has been reported associated with cocaine use and is thought to be secondary to the acute hypertension and vasoconstriction induced by cocaine.

In addition to the infective risks of intravenous drug users, the cocaine-abusing mother is at risk from many acute reactions (Table 6.2).

Adverse renal effects have been reported characterised by haematuria, proteinuria, haemolytic anaemia and renal insufficiency. Acute pulmonary oedema can occur, which may reflect transient left ventricular dysfunction or a direct pulmonary microcirculatory effect. Cocaine abuse can be confused with pre-eclampsia in its presentation, as hypertension is often a prominent feature. Thrombocytopaenia is well described.

Table 6.2 – Complications of cocaine abuse.

Arrhythmias
Coronary ischaemia and infarction
Intracerebral haemorrhage
Convulsions
Hepatic rupture
Spontaneous pneumothorax
Uterine rupture after previous Caesarean section

Amphetamines

Amphetamines are sympathomimetic drugs, which have abuse potential by virtue of their stimulant effect. Their use in pregnancy is not uncommon and will often be in association with other drugs. Clinical presentation is much the same as cocaine. They do not appear to cause foetal abnormalities but may be associated with intrauterine growth retardation and premature labour. Specific maternal effects, which are not confined to pregnancy, are hypertension, tachycardia and hyperthermia. The principles of management are very similar to those used for cocaine abusers.

Benzodiazepines

Benzodiazepines are one of the most commonly prescribed class of drugs in the UK and temazepam is especially easily to obtain. The effects on pregnancy are uncertain but the use of diazepam in early pregnancy has been associated with an increased incidence of cleft palate, and high doses may result in a syndrome of withdrawal in the neonate. Detoxification should be done slowly, as excessive rapid withdrawal can lead to maternal convulsions.

MANAGEMENT OPTIONS AND DISCUSSION

HIV status

There are clear benefits in screening for HIV infection during pregnancy as knowledge of status not only gives women the option of appropriate management of their infection, but also allows decisions to be made about methods to reduce the rate of neonatal transmission. The risk of transmission to the baby can be substantially reduced (to below 2%) with antiretroviral therapy, treatment of associated infections, elective Caesarean section before rupture of membranes and avoidance of breast-feeding.

Hepatitis screening

Antenatal screening for Hepatitis B carrier status will allow prevention of perinatal transmission by immunisation of the baby. There is no effective immunisation for Hepatitis C or intervention to prevent perinatal transmission.

Opioid use

Use of opioids can cause reduced foetal heart rate variability and consequently cause difficulties in the interpretation of the CTG. Reversal of maternal opioid intoxication with naloxone can precipitate foetal distress and similarly, reversal of neonatal sedation with naloxone can be dangerous causing acute neonatal withdrawal.

The woman's drug problem may be recognised for the first time in labour. Withdrawal from opioids in labour may be shown by foetal distress on the CTG, increased foetal movements or meconium-stained liquor. Maternal signs include restlessness, tremors, sweating, abdominal pain, cramps, anxiety and vomiting. Any drug user, who goes into opioid withdrawal during labour, should be treated with a small dose of opioid.

Pain relief in labour and after a Caesarean section

Drug-abusing patients may be uncooperative for a variety of reasons. They may be anxious about being in hospital, in pain, withdrawing from drugs or fear the negative attitudes of health care professionals. Perceptions are changing among the latter, with drug abuse and alcoholism being considered more of an illness than a moral weakness. It is important to maintain a positive and non-judgemental attitude towards the mother.

During the course of labour, all types of analgesia should be available. Opioids for pain management are not contraindicated and should be given as to any woman in labour; however, larger doses may be required. Epidural analgesia is often particularly appropriate, if there are no medical contraindications.

After a Caesarean section, patients who have not received spinal morphine or diamorphine as part of the anaesthetic technique for Caesarean section are usually given a PCA morphine device (with a bolus of 1 mg) and a lockout of 5 min. Opioid-dependent patients on prescribed methadone can also have PCA morphine at the standard dose. The bolus dose may be increased if found to be insufficient, as in our case. A 'contract' should be made with the mother that the device will only be used for 1–2 days, until she is able to take analgesia orally, as it is a standard practice in non-drug using mothers.

Other labour ward management issues

As in this case, venous access can be a major problem. Repeated non-sterile injection over years destroys peripheral veins, often leaving track marks (thrombosed, fibrosed veins). Usually, a small amount of blood can be obtained peripherally, with patience, asking the mother's advice about likely sites and using a small needle. If intravenous access is required in labour, it may be wise to set up an external jugular line electively, rather than wait until an emergency situation. If this is not successful, then central venous access may be necessary.

Obliterated arm veins may lead an injecting drug user to access the femoral vein or indeed the artery. Constant use of the femoral vein invariably leads to the formation of a deep vein thrombosis. Repeated puncture of the femoral artery may cause distal embolisation and aneursym formation requiring surgery.

Universal precautions should be employed for these patients. We should, of course, assume that every patient poses an innoculation risk as up to 40% of the population infected with HIV are unaware of the fact.

Specific management issues associated with cocaine abuse

Once identified, these women should be encouraged to stop using the drug. There are no effective pharmacological agents to block cocaine craving and to sustain abstinence. Acute intoxication with cocaine can be life-threatening at any point in gestation. Usually this is self-limiting and prolonged intoxication should raise suspicions of continued ingestion, for example body packing. Agitation and hypertension may resolve with benzodiazepines, but labetolol may be required to control hypertensive crises. Hyperthermia is treated symptomatically, and seizures may require benzodiazepine treatment.

In the presence of acute cocaine intoxication, non-emergency surgery should be delayed, but this may not be possible in the obstetric setting where recent ingestion may cause foetal distress or placental abruption.

Analgesia and anaesthesia

1. Regional anaesthesia in cocaine-abusing patients is associated with difficulties:
    (a) potentially uncooperative patient if acutely intoxicated;
    (b) vasoconstriction and reduced circulating volume may make epidural anaesthesia preferable to subarachnoid blockade;
    (c) indirectly acting vasoconstrictors, such as ephedrine, may be less effective in chronic cocaine abusers because of neurotransmitter depletion;
    (d) there is a potentially dangerous interaction with directly acting sympathomimetics causing tachycardia, hypertension, left ventricular failure and pulmonary oedema;
    (e) thrombocytopaenia.

2. Specific problems associated with general anaesthesia:
    (a) Hypertension at laryngoscopy, intubation and extubation may be a problem. The usual agents selected to attenuate these responses (i.e. alfentanil, fentanyl and labetolol) appear to be safe in the context of acute intoxication.

KEY LEARNING POINTS

1. With an increasing incidence of drug abuse in the UK, it is likely that as anaesthetists we will encounter these mothers more frequently on the delivery suite.

2. Opiates and benzodiazepines should not be stopped abruptly during pregnancy, but other illicit drugs should be discontinued as soon as possible.

3. Effective comprehensive care of drug-addicted women has been shown to improve maternal and neonatal outcomes. This hinges on a multidisciplinary approach, which addresses both medical and social issues.

4. The optimal time to discuss the management of pain relief in labour and after a Caesarean section is in an obstetric anaesthetic clinic. Clearly made plans will help reduce difficult, aggressive behaviour in the acute situation by removing the uncertainty about suitable methods of pain relief.

Further reading

Campbell D, Parr M, Shutt L. Unrecognised 'crack' cocaine abuse in pregnancy. *British Journal of Anaesthesia* 1996; **77**: 553–5.

Kandall S, Doberczak T, Jantunen M, *et al*. The methadone-maintained pregnancy. *Clinics in Perinatology* 1999; **26**: 173–83.

Livingston J, Mabie B, Ramanathan J. Crack cocaine, myocardial infarction, and Troponin I levels at the time of Caesarean delivery. *Anesthesia and Analgesia* 2000; **91**: 913–15.

Mandelbrot L, Le Chenadec J, Berrebi A, *et al*. Decreased perinatal HIV-1 transmission following elective caesarean delivery with zidovudine treatment. *JAMA* 1998; **280**: 55–60.

Mulleague L, Bonner SM, Samuel A, *et al*. Wound botulism in drug addicts in the United Kingdom. *Anaesthesia* 2001; **56**: 119–23.

Siney C. *Pregnancy and Drug Abuse*. Books for Midwives Press, Cheshire, 1999.

Singh P, Dimich I, Shamsi A. Intraoperative pulmonary oedema in a young cocaine smoker. *Canadian Journal of Anaesthesia* 1994; **41**: 961–4.

Sprauve ME. Substance abuse and HIV in pregnancy. *Clinical Obstetrics and Gynaecology* 1996; **39**: 316–30.

7

MASSIVE OBSTETRIC HAEMORRHAGE

J. Sewell

CASE HISTORY

A 34-year-old Caucasian woman, gravida 4, para 2, was admitted at 33 weeks gestation with a small, revealed, ante-partum bleed. She had a past history of frequent urinary tract infections (UTIs) and menorrhagia, and her obstetric history included a stillbirth at 23 weeks from hydrops foetalis, which had been delivered by emergency Caesarean section. She had two subsequent uneventful elective Caesareans under epidural anaesthesia.

This pregnancy had been complicated by some pain and blood loss in the first trimester and an ultrasound scan had shown a retroplacental clot, a low-lying anterolateral placenta and a baby with a cystic hygroma. On the day of admission, she had a small bleed but the cardiotocograph (CTG) was satisfactory and immediate delivery of the baby was not considered necessary; betamethasone was given. The following evening, she had a further bleed and it was decided to proceed to urgent Caesarean section.

In view of the history of ante-partum haemorrhage (APH), previous Caesarean section and a pre-operative haemoglobin of 10.6 g/dl, 6 units of blood were cross matched. The mother expressed a wish to be awake during the birth so a spinal anaesthetic was considered appropriate. No major problems were anticipated so an experienced staff grade obstetrician and an anaesthetic registrar started the case as it was after 5 p.m.

At operation, she was found to have a low, anterior placenta accreta, the baby was delivered rapidly in good condition but the patient then began to bleed profusely. Fortunately, despite it being around 9 p.m., a consultant obstetrician was on the premises and arrived within minutes of being called. The anaesthetist called for help from the resident second on call registrar and the duty consultant, who arrived from home in 20 min.

The patient became hypotensive despite rapid i.v. fluid replacement through two large bore cannulae with a blood warmer and began to lose consciousness, so general anaesthesia was induced. Central venous access was achieved with a Drum-cath in an antecubital fossa vein and an arterial line was inserted. The surgeons proceeded rapidly to hysterectomy, blood loss was estimated at 6 l, and blood taken during this time showed a haemoglobin of 4.4 g/dl, activated partial thromboplastin time (APTT) of 80 s with a ratio of 2.5. Prothrombin time (PT), international normalised ratio (INR) and fibrinogen were unmeasurable. Arterial pH was 7.2 with a base excess of −18 mmol/l, pCO_2 of 22 mmHg and pO_2 of 344 mmHg. In all, she received 3.7 l of crystalloid, 4.5 l of colloid, 10 units of packed red cells, 20 units of platelets, six of fresh frozen plasma (FFP) and 15 of cryoprecipitate. She was also given ephedrine, adrenaline, atropine and calcium chloride.

With surgery completed and bleeding controlled, the patient was transferred to the main intensive therapy unit (ITU). On arrival, her central venous pressure (CVP) was 8 cmH₂O, Hb 7.9 g/dl, platelets 148×10^9/l, INR 1.3, pH 7.22 and base excess −9 mmol/l. She made a full recovery, apart from needing a stent for a partially-obstructed ureter, and went home after 9 days. Her baby joined her after a fortnight in SCBU.

DESCRIPTION OF THE PROBLEM

Massive haemorrhage has been defined in various ways (e.g. the loss of more than half the circulating volume in 3 h, or 150 ml/min). However, blood loss is difficult to estimate at the best of times so a more useful working definition is major blood loss, which is difficult to control and requires the rapid transfusion of large volumes of fluid and red cells.

Haemorrhage, excluding early pregnancy bleeding due to ectopic pregnancy or miscarriage, is still the sixth commonest cause of maternal deaths in the UK and is due to placental abruption, placenta praevia or post-partum haemorrhage (PPH). In the 1997–9 triennial report, it was the direct cause of seven deaths, which was an improvement on the previous reports, but still gives a risk of about 1 in 100,000 maternities; this compares to 1 in 1000 in developing countries, where it is still by far the commonest cause of death. The risk of potentially life-threatening haemorrhage has been estimated as occurring in 1 in 1000 deliveries, or 600 per year in the UK. This equates to two or three major haemorrhages per year in an average maternity unit, making it a fairly rare but serious event that must be managed well on every occasion.

1.   For this reason, it is essential that all maternity units should have clearly displayed guidelines for managing major haemorrhage, and that all staff should be familiar with them and exposed to regular 'drills'.

2. Careful evaluation of each delivery may make it possible to anticipate some cases (e.g. placenta praevia, previous haemorrhage, multiple pregnancy, obesity, a large baby or advanced maternal age), but not all.

PATHOPHYSIOLOGY

Losing a mother from catastrophic haemorrhage is a devastating event for all concerned. The distress is compounded when care is sub-standard, which has been shown in many cases. Documented examples of sub-standard care include: management by insufficiently experienced staff, poor communication between labour ward and blood bank (including the two being on different sites), and accident and emergency staff not recognising the serious implications of apparently minor symptoms and signs in obstetric patients. This sub-standard care typically leads to delay in correction of hypovolaemia, delay in recognition of coagulation disorder and delay in surgical control of bleeding. While death from haemorrhage is rare, morbidity is not and includes hypovolaemic shock, poor foetal outcome (especially in the case of placental abruption), disseminated intravascular coagulation (DIC), acute respiratory distress syndrome (ARDS) and renal failure. Sheehans syndrome due to avascular necrosis of the anterior pituitary still occurs.

MANAGEMENT OPTIONS AND DISCUSSION

The outcome in this case was successful but nevertheless several useful lessons were learned. Foremost among these were: the importance of good communications, the presence of senior staff and the capacity to get large volumes of suitable blood to the delivery suite very quickly.

1. There had been some difficulty obtaining sufficient quantities of blood for two reasons. Firstly, her blood group was O negative and there were only seven units of O negative blood in the hospital. The regional Blood Transfusion Service is a short walk away from the hospital but it was necessary to call a taxi to fetch more blood supplies.

2. Secondly, there were communication difficulties between theatre and blood bank at the start of the crisis. These were resolved when a senior midwife set herself up as the sole link between the two, and moved bodily from one to the other transporting information and blood products.

MANAGEMENT OF MAJOR HAEMORRHAGE

Effective management of major haemorrhage starts with giving oxygen, then rapid infusion of crystalloids and red cells, after taking blood for cross match, full blood count (FBC), clotting screen and basic biochemistry. A proprietary blood warmer should be used (since hypothermia worsens clotting disorders), with an in-line 170 µm filter and if possible a rapid infuser device, such as Level 1 (Graseby) or

Ranger (Actamed). Outcome in critically-ill patients may be better if crystalloids, preferably Hartmann's solution, are used rather than colloids as large volumes of colloids can compound haemostatic disorders, but in this type of situation there must be a priority to restore circulating blood volume to prevent severe end-organ damage. Red cells are usually supplied as packed cells and group O negative, group specific or fully cross-matched blood can be given according to urgency. A full cross match should not take more than 30 min.

Monitoring of response is essential and involves from the start observation of conscious level, urine output, pulse, BP and foetal well-being if ante-partum. Blood loss of up to 1000 ml is well tolerated in late pregnancy and foetal distress on the CTG is a sensitive sign of maternal hypotension since perfusion to vital organs is maintained at the expense of uteroplacental blood flow. There should be very close monitoring of any mother who has an estimated blood loss of 1000–1500 ml as she may look well initially, but may physiologically decompensate rapidly. When haemorrhage becomes severe and on going, monitoring should include CVP, intra-arterial blood pressure measurement and blood gas and acid–base analysis.

When large volumes of fluid and packed cells are given, a coagulation disorder is likely to develop. This should be monitored by regular clotting studies, and FFP administered at a rate of 4 units for every 6 units of red cells if *clotting times are prolonged* and there is *continued bleeding*. Platelets will be needed if the transfusion exceeds about 1.5 times blood volume and cryoprecipitate if there are signs of DIC. This will be indicated by abnormal clotting tests despite FFP and a fibrinogen level less than 1 g/dl with raised levels of fibrin degradation products (FDP) and D-dimer.

While resuscitation is in progress, urgent attention should be given to treating the cause of the bleeding. In the case of major APH, delivery of the baby should be rapidly achieved by Caesarean section unless the baby is dead, in which case labour may be induced if the mother's condition is stable. With severe bleeding from placenta praevia, urgent Caesarean section is required and surgical control of bleeding may include ligation of the uterine or internal iliac arteries, or hysterectomy.

PPH is usually due to uterine atony and treatment requires exclusion of retained products or genital tract trauma, followed by administration of oxytocin and prostaglandin F2α analogues, such as carboprost (Hemabate). Occasionally, uterine packing or even hysterectomy may be needed.

Every maternity unit must have guidelines for managing massive haemorrhage, as suggested above, and they cannot be summarised better than by Prof. J. Bonnar's 'ORDER', given here in outline:

Organisation

1. Call consultant obstetrician, anaesthetist, haematologist and experienced midwife.

2. Alert blood bank technician.

3. One nurse appointed to record vital signs, urine output, fluids and drugs given.

4. One person appointed to liase with blood bank technician.

5. Operating theatre on standby.

Restoration of blood volume

1. 2 × 14 gauge IV cannulae.

2. Blood for cross matching 6 units, FBC, U&E, clotting screen.

3. Hartmann's solution rapidly infused with blood warmer.

4. If haemorrhage life threatening, give O negative blood.

5. Give ABO and rhesus D compatible blood as soon as possible.

Defective blood coagulation

1. Check platelet count, APTT and PT. If abnormal, check thrombin time, fibrinogen and D–dimers.

2. Prolonged clotting tests and oozing from puncture sites, give FFP.

3. If platelet count less than $50 \times 10^9/l$, give platelet concentrates.

4. If clotting tests not corrected by FFP and severe bleeding continues, give cryoprecipitate.

5. Before surgical intervention, give cryoprecipitate and platelets (ideally to platelet count more than $80 \times 10^9/l$ before starting).

6. The management of severe on going clotting problems can be improved by consultation with a haematologist.

Evaluation of response

1. Monitor pulse, BP, CVP, blood gases and acid–base status.

2. Urine output by indwelling catheter.

3. Regular Hb and haematocrit assessment, and clotting tests to guide the use of blood components.

Remedy the cause of bleeding

1. If APH, deliver the foetus and placenta.

2. If PPH, use oxytocin and prostaglandin.

3. Examine genital tract, explore uterine cavity, ligate bleeding vessels and consider uterine packing.

4. Ligation of uterine arteries, internal iliac and ovarian arteries.

5. Arterial embolisation.

6. Hysterectomy.

MANAGEMENT OF A JEHOVAH'S WITNESS

Jehovah's Witnesses who decline blood transfusion should be managed as follows: Firstly, it is even more important to anticipate major blood loss when risk factors are present, and senior staff should be informed when a Jehovah's Witness is admitted in labour. The 3rd stage of labour should be managed actively and a syntocinon infusion started immediately after delivery if any risk factors for PPH exist.

For active haemorrhage give crystalloids and colloids as above. Syntometrine may be more effective than syntocinon and early use of misoprostol and carboprost should be considered.

Drugs that have been used to reduce haemorrhage include aprotinin and tranexamic acid (both fibrinolytic inhibitors), which can be used in combination. More recently, recombinant factor VIIa has been used, although its use in obstetric haemorrhage has not been evaluated. If these drugs are to be considered, a senior haematologist must be involved in the decision-making process.

Surgical procedures to control bleeding should be performed by a consultant without delay. The B-Lynch brace suture may avoid the need for hysterectomy if used early before major coagulation disorders occur. Blood salvage by cell saver has been described and can be life saving if the mother refuses stored blood. With the normal washing process and the use of leucocyte depletion filters, amniotic fluid and foetal squames cells are removed.

In the recovery phase of a major haemorrhage with severe anaemia, erythropoietin and IV iron sucrose and hyperbaric oxygen have been described.

KEY LEARNING POINTS

1. Massive obstetric haemorrhage is common in the UK but occurs only occasionally in an individual maternity unit.

2. The outcome can be devastating but a successful outcome is more likely if cases are anticipated, senior staff are involved, volume replacement is prompt and aggressive, and large volumes of suitable blood and blood products are rapidly available.

3. All maternity units must have up-to-date guidelines on the management of major haemorrhage and they should be regularly tested to iron out local difficulties in their implementation.

Further reading

B-Lynch C, Coker A, Lawal AH, Abu J, Cowen MJ. The B-Lynch surgical technique for the control of massive postpartum haemorrhage: an alternative to hysterectomy? Five cases reported. *British Journal of Obstetrics and Gynaecology* 1997; **104**: 372–5.

Bonnar J. Order for management of massive obstetric haemorrhage. *Best Practice and Research in Clinical Obstetrics and Gynaecology* **14**: 6–15.

Busuttil D, Copplestone A. Management of blood loss in Jehovah's Witnesses. *British Medical Journal* 1995; **311**: 115–16.

Catling SJ, Freites S, Krishnan S, Gibbs R. Clinical experience with cell salvage in obstetrics: 4 cases from one UK centre. *International Journal of Obstetric Anesthesia* 2002; **11**: 128–34.

Hewitt PE, Machin SJ. Massive blood transfusion. In *ABC of Transfusion*. BMJ Publishing Group, London, 1998, pp. 49–52.

Mantel C, Buchmann E, Rees H, Pattinson RC. Severe acute maternal morbidity: a pilot study of a definition for a near miss. *British Journal of Obstetrics and Gynaecology* 1998; **105**: 985–90.

McClelland DBL (ed.). Optimal use of donor blood. *Report from a Working Party set up by the Clinical Resource and Audit Group.* The Scottish Office, Edinburgh, 1995.

Why mothers die 1997–1999. *Report on Confidential Enquiries into Maternal Deaths in the UK.* RCOG press, London, 2001.

8

ISCHAEMIC HEART DISEASE IN PREGNANCY

C. Egeler and M.J. Evans

CASE HISTORY

A 38-year-old multigravida presented to the A/E department at 16 weeks gestation with a 1-h history of central chest pain radiating to her left arm accompanied with breathlessness and nausea. She was a heavy smoker of 20 pack years, overweight with a body mass index of $30 \, kg/m^2$ and there was a positive family history of ischaemic heart disease. She had been on oral contraceptives until 2 years ago and since had a normal delivery following an uncomplicated pregnancy. She took no medication but admitted to the occasional use of ecstasy and cocaine. On examination, she was in pain, blood pressure was 190/90 mmHg with a pulse rate of 110 beats/min and there was a grade 2, non-radiating, systolic murmur over the aortic area. An ECG showed sinus rhythm with ST depression of 3 mm over the antero-lateral leads.

Her symptoms improved with the use of nitrates, diamorphine and meto-clopramide. ECG changes disappeared and subsequent cardiac enzymes and troponin-T levels were within normal limits although cholesterol and triglyceride levels were found to be increased. She was started on atenolol 50 mg daily and aspirin 75 mg and was strongly advised to stop smoking. A coronary angiogram performed at 25 weeks gestation showed atheromatous changes resulting in a 75% occlusion in the left anterior descending artery and minor changes in the right circumflex artery. In an exercise tolerance test, she reached a workload of 50 W/min at which point, the test had to be terminated because of exhaustion. Heart rate was 138 beats/min and minor ST depression over the anterolateral leads was present. Her medication was continued and she was seen at regular intervals in both the obstetric and cardiology outpatient clinic. No further episodes of chest pain occurred, although she continued to smoke.

At 37 weeks gestation, she presented with elevated blood pressure and proteinuria. She was breathless on mild exertion but had no chest pain. ECG showed sinus rhythm with a lateral strain pattern. The baby appeared to be small for gestation but healthy on ultrasound scan. After a multidisciplinary discussion, it was decided to induce labour.

Continuous ECG, pulse oximetry plus non-invasive blood pressure monitoring were used as well as routine cardiotocography (CTG). Since oxygen saturation was only 94% on air, oxygen 2 l/min was administered via a nasal cannula, resulting in an increase in saturation to 99%. A lumbar epidural catheter was inserted without difficulty and, using incremental bolus doses of 5 ml of 0.2% plain bupivacaine with fentanyl 10 μg/ml, a block level to T10 bilaterally was achieved resulting in good analgesia and stable cardiovascular parameters. A continuous infusion of 0.15% bupivacaine with 2 μg/ml fentanyl was then started.

During the first few hours of labour, the patient remained cardiovascularly stable with good analgesia and a reactive CTG. She progressed to 5-cm dilatation when her blood pressure rose to 170/100 mmHg and the patient began complaining of chest tightness and increased shortness of breath. A repeat 12-lead ECG showed mild ST depression anterolaterally and she was commenced on a GTN infusion, which improved her symptoms. It was decided to commence invasive monitoring and an arterial cannula was inserted in her left radial artery and a central venous line through the right internal jugular vein under aseptic precautions. Central venous pressure (CVP) was 12 mmHg but transiently rose by 2–10 mmHg during each contraction.

Three hours later, she was found to be fully dilated and an episiotomy was performed to facilitate a high cavity forceps extraction of a healthy 2860-g boy with Apgar scores of 9 and 10 at 1 and 5 min, respectively. Active expulsions were not allowed during delivery. Shortly after administration of 5 IU oxytocin, she complained of breathlessness and her oxygen saturation decreased to 92%. Her CVP measured 18 mmHg and she was found to have fine crepitations in both lung bases on auscultation. Frusemide 20 mg was given resulting in a good diuresis, a decrease in her CVP and improvement of her oxygenation. The patient remained closely monitored for 48 h in a high dependency setting during which she had no further complications.

DESCRIPTION OF THE PROBLEM

1. Ischaemic heart disease is still a rare condition in women of childbearing age.

2. The physiological changes that occur during pregnancy and labour markedly increase cardiac workload and oxygen requirements. If oxygen demand cannot be met by supply, ischaemia will result.

3. Women with symptoms or a history of ischaemic heart disease require special consideration and careful multidisciplinary management during pregnancy and labour.

PATHOPHYSIOLOGY

The changes in cardiovascular parameters during pregnancy and labour are well recognised. In the first trimester, plasma volume will increase by 20% and by the end of the second trimester, red cell mass will have risen by 20% along with a 45% rise in plasma volume. This results in a 50% increase in cardiac output, which is achieved through a 25% increase in stroke volume and heart rate.

During labour, cardiac output increases by a further 15% during the latent phase, 30% during the active phase and up to 45% during the expulsive phase. Ueland reported an increase in cardiac workload up to 80% during expulsion under local anaesthesia only. Less dramatic changes are observed when conduction blockade is used, which implies that pain is a major determinant of cardiovascular stress during labour. In addition, 300–500 ml uterine blood enters the maternal circulation and increases preload during each contraction. It has been demonstrated that this pushes the CVP up by 5–20 mmHg.

These changes represent a considerable workload for the myocardium, which will in turn have a considerably higher oxygen demand. Oxygen extraction from the myocardium in pregnancy is already 70–80% at rest and any increased demand can only be met by an increase in blood flow to the coronary arteries. Oxygen extraction only occurs during diastole (particularly for the left ventricle) and is dependent on pulse rate. In addition, a high ventricular wall tension caused by increased ventricular filling depresses blood flow to the subendocardium, which will be the first area to become hypoxic. Any constriction in coronary blood flow, such as sclerosis or thrombosis, may therefore significantly impair oxygen supply to the myocardium rendering it ischaemic and at worst cause myocardial infarction.

A further risk factor that may reduce coronary artery flow or cause obstruction lies in the hypercoagulable state of pregnancy. Although coagulation tests remain normal, higher levels of fibrinogen, and clotting factors VII, VIII, IX, X and XII are found.

The incidence of ischaemic heart disease in pregnancy is generally estimated to be 1 : 1000. Risk factors include positive family history, oral contraceptives (which may alter the lipid profile and predispose to thrombosis), obesity, diabetes and hyper-lipidaemia. Lifestyle also plays an important role as many women nowadays postpone childbearing until later in life to pursue a professional career. This may result in higher stress levels and increased use of recreational drugs and smoking. Smoking alone increases the risk of myocardial infarction by a factor of three, compared to non-smoking pre-menopausal women. The abuse of drugs, such as cocaine, has also been linked to premature atherosclerosis and may lead to myocardial infarction as a result of coronary artery spasm or thrombotic events.

Myocardial infarction in pregnancy was first described in 1922 and about 100 cases have since been reported. It has been calculated that 1 out of 10 myocardial infarctions in women under 50 years of age occur in the peri-partum period. In the Report on Confidential Enquiries into Maternal Deaths in the UK over the period from 1994–1996, there were six deaths due to myocardial infarction, and in the Report 1997–1999, there were a further five deaths. Hankins *et al.* reviewed 68 published cases of myocardial infarction during pregnancy of which only 13% of mothers were known to have ischaemic heart disease before they became pregnant. Of infarctions 13% occurred in the first, 25% in the second and 62% in the third trimesters of pregnancy. Maternal mortality was 11%, 29% and 45%, respectively, which emphasises the need for identifying women at risk as early as possible in pregnancy. This, however, remains as a difficult task as often there are no preceding symptoms of ischaemic heart disease.

The underlying pathological mechanisms are coronary artery spasm (which may be the result of renin release from a transiently ischaemic chorion), embolic events (either from the placenta or caused by the hypercoagulable state of pregnancy), spontaneous coronary artery dissection, pre-eclampsia and use of oxytocic drugs. The anterior descending artery was most commonly involved leading to an impairment of anterior ventricular wall function.

MANAGEMENT OPTIONS AND DISCUSSION

General plan

The management of a pregnant patient with ischaemic heart disease has to take a multidisciplinary approach involving the cardiologist, obstetrician and anaesthetist in the decision-making process. During pregnancy, hospitalisation may be required to ensure adequate rest to minimise myocardial oxygen consumption. The decision to induce labour is usually founded on obstetric indications. Labour within 2 weeks of infarction carries the poorest prognosis. There is debate about whether Caesarean section should be the preferred method of delivery. The advantages include having a more controlled situation and a quick delivery, as well as avoidance of cardiovascular stress during labour. Hankins, however, found a maternal mortality following myocardial infarction of 23% after Caesarean section compared to 14% after vaginal delivery, although this difference might be accounted for by different patient characteristics. Ginz reported that mortality was nil for those delivered by forceps compared to 13% for non-interventional delivery and 27% for Caesarean section. It has also been shown that cardiac output may increase up to 50% during Caesarean section under subarachnoid block. Too few reports exist to make a definite case for or against Caesarean section and at present the decision for operative delivery in a stable patient is based on obstetric indications.

Analgesia and anaesthesia

Both general and regional anaesthesia have been used successfully for operative delivery.

General anaesthesia carries the well-acknowledged risk of airway control in a mother who is often obese and smokes. Induction and intubation with standard general anaesthetic drugs for Caesarean section may also cause an undesired sympathetic response. A well-conducted general anaesthetic will, however, reduce myocardial oxygen demand while ensuring optimum oxygenation if sympathetic blockade is undesirable.

Regional anaesthesia may be an epidural, combined spinal–epidural or spinal catheter technique depending on the patient's cardiovascular stability, coagulation profile and operator experience. All regional techniques should consist of carefully titrated block set against the cardiovascular response.

Administration of supplementary oxygen and continuous monitoring of the cardiovascular system and oxygenation is mandatory for both vaginal and operative delivery but the additional use of invasive lines including a pulmonary artery floatation catheter should always be considered to aid management.

Conduction blockade is definitely indicated in labour to limit pain-induced cardiovascular stress and the resultant vasodilatation may be helpful, but additional use of parenteral nitrates might be required to further reduce preload. Loop diuretics are indicated if there are signs of left ventricular failure in the acute situation. The judicious use of synthetic oxytocic drugs after delivery will minimise sudden increases in preload due to uterine blood entering the maternal circulation while ensuring adequate uterine contraction. Syntocinon 5 units given slowly is the drug of choice.

Following delivery, it is essential to continue close monitoring to avoid adverse events in the post-partum period and it may be appropriate to care for the mother on a coronary care unit.

KEY LEARNING POINTS

1. Ischaemic heart disease in pregnancy remains a rare encounter but may potentially be disastrous for the patient if not managed properly.

2. Early multidisciplinary management is essential with clearly written plans for the anaesthetic management of delivery.

3. Continuous non-invasive monitoring during labour is mandatory and invasive lines should be considered early.

4. Epidural analgesia, a short spontaneous labour and assisted delivery without active expulsion seem to carry the least mortality, while Caesarean section is usually indicated for obstetric reasons.

5. Oxytocic drugs cause haemodynamic instability and can cause a sudden increase in cardiac-filling pressures, which may precipitate pulmonary oedema. These drugs must be given with caution and by infusion rather than as a large bolus.

Further reading

Aglio LS, Johnson MD. Anaesthetic management of myocardial infarction in a parturient. *British Journal of Anaesthesia* 1990; **65**: 139–46.

Bonica JJ. Maternal anatomic and physiological alterations during pregnancy and parturition. In: Bonica JJ, Mcdonald JS (eds) *Principles and Practice of Obstetric Analgesia*. Williams and Wilkins, Baltimore, 1995, pp. 45–83.

Croft P, Hannaford PC. Risk factors for acute myocardial infarction in women: evidence from the Royal College of General Practitioners' oral contraceptive study. *British Medical Journal* 1989; **298**: 165–8.

Fletcher AP, Alkjaersig NK, Burstein R. The influence of pregnancy upon blood coagulation and plasma fibrinolytic enzyme function. *American Journal of Obstetrics and Gynecology* 1979; **134**: 743–51.

Frenkel Y, Barkai G, Reisin L, *et al*. Pregnancy after myocardial infarction: are we playing safe? *Obstetrics and Gynaecology* 1991; **77**: 822–5.

Ginz B. Myocardial infarction in pregnancy. *The Journal of Obstetrics and Gynaecology of the British Commonwealth* 1970; **77**: 610–15.

Hankins GDV, Wendel GD, Leveno KL, Stoneham J. Myocardial infarction during pregnancy: a review. *Obstetrics and Gynaecology* 1985; **65**: 139–46.

Hendricks CH. The haemodynamics of a uterine contraction. *American Journal of Obstetrics and Gynecology* 1938; **76**: 969.

Jackson G. Coronary artery disease and women. *British Medical Journal* 1994; **309**: 555–6.

Lees MM, Taylor SH, Scott DB, *et al.* A study of cardiac output at rest throughout pregnancy. *Journal of Obstetrics and Gynaecology of the British Commonwealth* 1967; **74**: 319.

Liu SS, Forrester RM, Murphy GS, *et al.* Anaesthetic management of a parturient with myocardial infarction related to cocaine use. *Canadian Journal of Anaesthesia* 1992; **39**: 858–61.

Mabie WC, Anderson GD, Addington MB, *et al.* The benefit of cesarean section in acute myocardial infarction complicated by premature labor. *Obstetrics and Gynaecology* 1988; **71**: 503–6.

Why mothers die. Report on Confidential Enquiries into Maternal Deaths in the United Kingdom, 1994–1996. London: The Stationery office, 1998, pp. 104–14.

Santos GS, Sadaniantz A. Postpartum acute myocardial infarction. *American Journal of Obstetrics and Gynecology* 1997; **177**: 1553–5.

Skinner SL, Lumbers ER, Symonds EM. Renin concentrations in human fetal and maternal tissues. *American Journal of Obstetrics and Gynecology* 1968; **101**: 529–33.

Söderlin MK, Purhonen S, Haring P, *et al.* Myocardial infarction in a parturient. *Anaesthesia* 1994; **49**: 870–2.

Ueland K, Gills RL, Hansen JM. Maternal cardiovascular dynamics. I. Cesarean section under subarachnoid block anesthesia. *American Journal of Obstetrics and Gynecology* 1968; **103**: 42.

Ueland K, Hansen JM. Maternal cardiovascular dynamics. II. Posture and uterine contractions. *American Journal of Obstetrics and Gynecology* 1969a; **103**: 1–7.

Ueland K, Hansen JM. Maternal cardiovascular dynamics III. Labour and delivery under local and caudal analgesia. *American Journal of Obstetrics and Gynecology* 1969; **103**: 8.

9

THE PREGNANT JEHOVAH'S WITNESS

S. Catling

CASE HISTORY

A 22-year-old gravida 1, Jehovah's Witness was seen at 12 weeks gestation with a history of anaemia. She was taking regular folic acid and her haematological profile at that time was normal (Table 9.1). She was seen by her consultant obstetrician the same week, and her wishes regarding refusal of blood and all blood products were clearly documented in the notes, along with all appropriately signed legal forms. Active management of the third stage of labour and the use of oxytocin were discussed and she was reassured that her decisions would be respected. By 30 weeks, she had developed significant anaemia, with a decrease in haemoglobin (Hb) concentration to 8.3 g/dl and haematocrit (Hct) of 0.25, and was started on oral ferrous sulphate 400 mg/day by her general practitioner. At the hospital antenatal clinic, she was thought to have polyhydramnios with a 'big baby' and gestational diabetes. Ultrasound scans confirmed a fundal placenta with a slightly increased liquor volume. Her serum ferritin was found to be low at 7 ng/ml (normal 10–300 ng/ml). There was an initial response to oral iron, but this was not sustained, despite increasing the dose to 600 mg/day, and at 37 weeks gestation her Hb remained low at 8.6 g/dl with Hct of 0.27. A hypochromic, microcytic blood film with a borderline low ferritin (11 ng/ml) suggested refractory, iron-deficiency anaemia, and she was admitted as an inpatient for parenteral iron therapy and rest. She looked pale and was breathless but not in cardiac failure. She was started on intramuscular iron sorbitol (Jectofer) 100 mg/day after discussion with the consultant haematologist. Two days later, she ruptured her membranes and went into spontaneous labour, which progressed normally to full dilatation of the cervix in 5 h, after which there was no further progress. She was diagnosed as 'failure to progress' after 2 h, with the foetal head arrested at the level of the ischial spines in the occipito-transverse position.

At this point, the duty anaesthetist was asked to provide analgesia for vaginal examination and trial of ventouse-assisted delivery with the possibility of proceeding to Caesarean section. The obstetric anaesthetists had not been previously consulted about this patient. The patient agreed to accept the technique of autologous transfusion by cell salvage provided the blood remained in continuity with her circulation, and the Haemonetics Cell Saver 5 was brought urgently to the obstetric theatre.

Spinal anaesthesia was established using 0.5% hyperbaric bupivacaine 2.6 ml and morphine 100 μg, which achieved an anaesthetic block to T4 bilaterally. The cell saver was primed with saline, so that the retransfusion bag contained 200 ml, and this was connected via a standard intravenous giving set to a 16G peripheral venous cannula (Figure 9.1). Vaginal examination confirmed transverse arrest of the foetal head at the level of the ischial spines with marked caput and moulding and a decision was made to proceed to Caesarean section.

The operation was technically difficult, and the initial uterine incision had to be extended laterally to permit delivery of the 4700 g foetus. Blood was aspirated to the cell-saver circuit as soon as delivery of baby and placenta was complete. Total blood loss was 1000 ml, and she received 1500 ml of Hartmann's solution during the procedure, as well as 6 mg of ephedrine to maintain her blood pressure. The patient remained comfortable throughout, and her blood pressure, pulse and oxygen saturation were satisfactory. Two 5-unit boluses of syntocinon at delivery were followed by an intravenous infusion of syntocinon 20 units in 500 ml saline. Approximately 250 ml of concentrated red cells, Hct 0.6, were retransfused by the end of surgery, representing a replaced blood loss of approximately 500 ml.

Her immediate post-operative Hb was 6.4 g/dl with Hct of 0.2 (Table 9.1), which decreased to a low of 6.1 g/dl on the 3rd day. She left hospital on the 4th day feeling tired but well, and continued to receive iron supplements for 6 weeks.

DEFINITION OF THE PROBLEM

'Every moving thing that liveth shall be meat for you; even as the green herb have I given you all things. But flesh with the life thereof, which is the blood thereof, shall ye not eat' (Genesis Chapter 9, verses 3–4). Based on the literal interpretation of this and similar biblical passages, most Jehovah's Witnesses refuse transfusion of blood and blood products.

Table 9.1 – Haematological results during pregnancy and delivery.

	Booking						1 day post-operative	3 days post-operative
	12/40	30/40	34/40	36/40	37/40	38/40		
Hb (g/dl)	12.0	8.3	9.3	9.2	8.6	9.1	6.4	6.1
White cell count ($\times 10^9$/l)	6.8	9.3	9.0	8.1	8.0	9.9	13.1	7.6
Platelets ($\times 10^9$/l)	192	215	169	187	172	192	172	279
MCV (fl)	85.7	80.4	76.6	75.5	74.4	76.5	76.9	81.0
MCH (pg)	30.3	26.2	26.2	24.9	23.6	24.5	24.4	
MCHC (g/dl)	35.4	32.5	34.1	32.9	31.7	32.1	31.7	
Hct	0.34	0.25	0.27	0.28	0.27	0.28	0.20	
Red blood cell ($\times 10^{12}$/l)	3.96	3.18	3.5	3.71	3.65	3.69	2.61	
Ferritin (ng/ml)			7		11			
Action taken		Oral FeSO$_4$ 400 mg	Oral FeSO$_4$ 600 mg	Admitted intra mus-cular – iron sorbitol 100 mg	Spon-taneous labour Em C/S	Having received cell-saver blood		

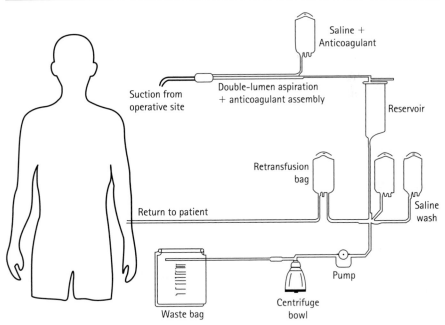

Saline + Anticoagulant

Double-lumen aspiration + anticoagulant assembly

Suction from operative site

Reservoir

Retransfusion bag

Return to patient

Saline wash

Pump

Waste bag

Centrifuge bowl

Figure 9.1 – Cell saver set up in continuity with circulation.

For elective surgery, mortality is hardly increased in Jehovah's Witnesses, and most problems arise in emergency cases with massive haemorrhage. Unfortunately, in obstetrics, massive haemorrhage is not uncommon, and the maternal death rate from haemorrhage remains at around 5.5 per million maternities. The 1991–1993 Triennial Report on Confidential Enquiries into Maternal Deaths in the UK, contains an appendix devoted to the problem of Jehovah's Witnesses, and highlights the fact that of the 15 deaths from haemorrhage, three had occurred in Jehovah's Witnesses. This represents a maternal death rate from haemorrhage of 1 in 1000, compared to less than 1 in 100,000 for the general maternity population.

PATHOPHYSIOLOGY

Tissue oxygenation starts to decline in most people when the Hb falls acutely below 7 g/dl. The degree to which Hb can fall and the patient still survives is uncertain. There are anecdotal accounts of patients surviving with Hb of around 2 g/dl. However, in any one individual, critical tissue oxygen delivery may be affected by factors such as concurrent disease and infection, but survival at Hb levels of 3–5 g/dl with general intensive care management is not uncommon, and only very exceptional cases survive at levels below this.

MANAGEMENT OPTIONS AND DISCUSSION

Antenatal planning

Jehovah's Witnesses should be identified at the booking visit and given the opportunity for a full discussion with the consultant obstetrician responsible for her care, so that it can be established clearly which treatments are to be avoided. There is variation among Jehovah's Witnesses about which blood fractions they will accept; some will accept none, while others may permit platelets, coagulation factors or albumin. Some will accept cell salvage, others have heard of 'artificial blood' or hyperbaric oxygen chambers, which they may believe are available to them on demand. In an emergency, there is no time for further exploration of the patient's wishes, so that clear documentation in the notes at this stage is vital.

The plan must be acceptable to all parties. If an individual clinician is not prepared to undertake responsibility for patients who are receiving 'substandard care – by their own choice', then care must be passed to a colleague willing to do so. Most areas have a local Hospital Liaison Committee, whose representatives are fully informed and prepared to help with communication and information problems.

It is essential that Jehovah's Witnesses are seen by a consultant obstetric anaesthetist at an early stage to determine what technical facilities are available locally and are acceptable to those involved. It is also important that Jehovah's Witnesses are treated by staff who are not antagonistic to their views. Attempts to argue with their views are ineffective and counter-productive and may interfere with the doctor–patient relationship. It is a criminal offence to transfuse blood without the patient's consent, and this should never be contemplated in any circumstances if the patient is a competent adult whose wishes are known.

Optimisation of haematocrit

Iron-deficiency anaemia in pregnancy is common and should be treated aggressively. However, simply starting the patient on oral iron tablets may not be effective, and early liaison with the haematologists to establish serum ferritin levels and body iron stores may be necessary. In our patient, even higher doses of oral iron (600 mg/day) were insufficient to restore her Hb to normal levels. Every effort should be made to bring these patients to term with a normal, or even slightly elevated Hb.

Erythropoietin

Erythropoietin (EPO) is a glycoprotein hormone which is the principal regulator of erythropoiesis. Recombinant human erythropoietin (rHuEPO) is manufactured from hamster ovary cells and is acceptable to Jehovah's Witnesses in the non-albumin-containing formulation (NeoRecormon, Epoetin beta, Roche). It has been studied extensively in patients with refractory anaemia associated with renal failure, and recent work has focused on its use as potential maternal therapy in various disorders of pregnancy, for example severe iron-deficiency anaemia, β-thalassaemia, and to increase Hb levels in patients wishing to donate autologous blood before elective surgery. EPO is an effective and safe stimulant to the differentiation of pluripotential stem cells into erythrocytes. It does not cross the placenta, and no anti-EPO antibodies have been detected, even after prolonged treatment. The hypertension occasionally seen in renal patients treated with rHuEPO seems not to occur in the non-renal population, and the only reported side effects are flu-like symptoms. The reticulocyte response may be limited by iron availability; so close monitoring of Hb and Hct is mandatory, with estimation of serum iron, iron-binding capacity and serum ferritin. The treatment appears safe in pregnant anaemic patients with no maternal, foetal or neonatal side effects. The recommended starting dose of rHuEPO is 60–80 units/kg weekly in divided doses three times per week by subcutaneous injection; increasing in steps of 20 units according to response. The aim should be to increase the Hb at a rate of up to 2 g/dl/month up to 10–12 g/dl. This treatment is expensive and the estimated UK cost for an 80-kg patient is between £160–500/week. This must be balanced against the potential cost of a prolonged stay on intensive therapy unit (ITU) following haemorrhage, if the Hb falls below the critical level needed for tissue oxygenation. A Jehovah's Witness patient with refractory anaemia and risk factors for haemorrhage could reasonably be given a trial of rHuEPO.

Identification of risk factors for haemorrhage

Successive Confidential Enquiries into Maternal Deaths have shown that postpartum haemorrhage occurs in about 1% of deliveries, and life-threatening haemorrhage occurs in about 1 in 1000 deliveries. Placenta praevia in patients with a uterine scar is a predictable cause of severe haemorrhage and increasing maternal age is a significant predisposing factor, especially if maternal age is greater than 35 years. High parity, pre-eclampsia, coagulation abnormalities and multiple pregnancy are all predictive factors for haemorrhage and these should be identified as early as possible and their increased significance in a Jehovah's Witness should be emphasised to patient and staff alike.

Methods of minimising operative blood loss

Surgery should be undertaken by the most experienced operator available, who not only should be able to perform Caesarean hysterectomy, but also should be sufficiently senior to make that decision rapidly. Carboprost (Hemabate, Pharmacia) 250 μg can be given by deep intramuscular injection for uterine atony refractory to ergometrine and oxytocin, and can be repeated at intervals of 15 min up to a total dose of 2 mg. There are three other types of pharmacological agents used in non-obstetric surgery to decrease blood loss: aprotinin (Trasylol, Bayer) a polypeptide, which inhibits proteolytic enzymes (such as plasmin and kallikrein); lysine analogues (such as amino-caproic acid and tranexamic acid (Cyklokapron, Pharmacia)), which are potent inhibitors of fibrinolysis; and desmopressin (DDAVP), a vasopressin analogue that leads to potentiation of primary haemostasis through an effect on coagulation factors. These agents have been studied extensively in cardiac surgery. Aprotinin and lysine analogues can significantly reduce operative blood loss and the need for transfusion in these circumstances, but the effect of desmopressin is minimal. There is little experience of the use of these agents in obstetrics, but on general principles they should have a beneficial effect in haemostasis. All such agents carry a risk of increased incidence of thrombosis.

Red cell–sparing techniques

In acute normovolaemic haemodilution, 2–3 units of blood (450 ml each) are removed from the circulation into blood-donation bags that remain in physical continuity with the circulation using three-way taps, with simultaneous volume replacement using crystalloid or colloid solutions to maintain normovolaemia. Blood removal can be achieved either via a central vein or a peripheral artery and may be useful in elective surgery with an anticipated blood loss exceeding 50% of estimated blood volume, provided the patient has a high initial Hct. Target Hct should be 25–30%, but mathematical modelling studies suggest that red cell sparing will be small. At the end of surgery, the 'removed' units are retransfused, either by simply opening the three-way tap and elevating the bag if a central vein was used, or via a pre-primed circuit to a peripheral vein if an artery was used.

The technique may improve oxygen delivery secondary to reduction in blood viscosity, and confers the benefit of returning blood containing normal concentrations of coagulation factors and functioning platelets at the end of the procedure.

It should only be considered if the pre-operative Hb is greater than 11 g/dl, and is inadvisable in the presence of myocardial ischaemia. It is not a licensed technique for pregnant patients, but is acceptable to many Jehovah's Witnesses and could be valuable for elective Caesarean section in a non-anaemic, fit Jehovah's Witness undergoing operation for conditions, such as placenta praevia with a risk of placenta percreta.

Red cell salvage

This technique suctions blood from the operative field and separates the red cells by centrifugation. After washing, the cells are resuspended in saline, filtered and ready for retransfusion within 3–5 min. The technique has wide applications in non-obstetric surgery, but is controversial in obstetrics because of the theoretical risk of incomplete removal of amniotic fluid from the blood for retransfusion, resulting in iatrogenic amniotic fluid embolism (AFE). The elements responsible for AFE are still not positively identified, but using the Haemonetics Cell Saver Five machine combined with the new generation leucocyte depletion filters (Pall RS, Pall Biomedical, Portsmouth, UK), it is now possible to demonstrate the complete removal of all protein and particulate elements studied so far. The cell saver is often acceptable to Jehovah's Witnesses as long as it is set up 'in continuity' with the circulation, which means priming all lines and the retransfusion bag with saline and connecting it to an indwelling intravenous cannula before the circuit is completed by suctioning blood from the operative site. Cell salvage should not begin until after delivery of the baby and placenta in order to reduce the initial amniotic fluid contamination of the salvaged blood. About 300 obstetric patients worldwide have been given cell-saved blood at Caesarean section, and there has been one reported death in a Jehovah's Witness with severe pre-eclampsia complicated by HELLP syndrome (haemolysis, elevated liver enzymes, low platelets) who was severely ill prior to retransfusion.

The cell saver can be set up in 5 min by an anaesthetic assistant and is simple to operate. In our case, we estimate that without the cell saver our patient's post-Caesarean Hb would have been approximately 4 g/dl, a figure at which tissue oxygenation may well have been critically impaired.

Unlike the haemodilution technique, cell salvage is applicable to emergency obstetric haemorrhage, even when the patient is anaemic beforehand, and is, therefore, of more practical value in the labour ward. The risks of iatrogenic AFE must be balanced against the consequences of letting the Hb fall to critical levels. It is an advantage for the patient to remain conscious throughout the procedure, so that she can be consulted about transfusion of homologous or cell-saved blood if the clinical situation deteriorates.

Red cell substitutes

The search continues for a safe and effective red cell substitute that will deliver oxygen as well as expand the circulating volume. Perfluorochemicals are synthetic, inert hydrophobic molecules with an unlimited capacity to dissolve oxygen. Although these fluids are cheap and easy to manufacture, they have a short half-life and require refrigerated storage, and are only effective when the patient breathes a high-inspired oxygen concentration. Fluosol DA did not fulfil early promise and is of no physiological benefit in severe anaemias. Newer preparations using smaller emulsion particles have been shown to have fewer side effects and may be more useful.

Hb-based oxygen carriers are also being studied and include recombinant Hb molecules, which may be acceptable to Jehovah's Witnesses. Hb in solution is vulnerable to oxidative inactivation, and to overcome this problem there are attempts to produce liposomal-encapsulated Hb solutions.

Mathematical modelling predicts that these solutions would be most effective in patients without pre-existing anaemia who undergo extreme haemodilution and lose large amounts of blood peri-operatively. If the problem of short half-life can be solved, these formulations may be extremely useful in massive haemorrhage in Jehovah's Witnesses. Although they are at present unlicensed, their use should be considered in patients in whom critical oxygen debt cannot be treated by other means.

Hyperbaric oxygen

With a physiological Hb of 15 g/dl, a PaO_2 of 12.0 kPa and normally functioning Hb, the Hb is 96.5% saturated. Each 100 ml of blood carries 19.68 ml of oxygen of which 0.28 ml is dissolved in plasma and 19.4 ml bound to Hb. If the Hb concentration is suddenly reduced to 3 g/dl, the total amount of oxygen carried per 100 ml blood is reduced to 4.16 ml. However, the amount of oxygen dissolved in plasma in physical solution obeys Henry's law and the content may be increased to useful values by hyperbaric oxygen therapy. At 3 atmospheres absolute (ATA) of 100% oxygen, the physically dissolved oxygen can supply the body's basic metabolic needs. However, acute oxygen toxicity occurs at above 1.8 ATA and is dose/time dependent, manifesting as central nervous system (CNS) toxicity with convulsions. Subacute oxygen toxicity also occurs at pressures above 0.5 ATA, requiring longer exposure and producing acute lung injury. Formulae exist for predicting likely toxic effects from any given exposure to hyperbaric oxygen in terms of pressure and time.

Intermittent hyperbaric oxygen therapy has been used in patients with severe post-haemorrhage anaemia and persistent lactic acidosis from anaerobic tissue metabolism. It is logistically difficult, but can improve tissue oxygenation until the anaemia improves under EPO therapy. The availability of such a treatment will depend on the geographical proximity of the intensive care unit to a hyperbaric unit able to adequately cope with a patient undergoing intensive care.

KEY LEARNING POINTS

1. Prevention is better than cure.

2. In the present situation of unlicensed red cell substitutes and the impracticality of hyperbaric oxygen therapy, patients with Hb less than 3.0 g/dl are unlikely to survive the critical oxygen debt even with prolonged intensive care.

3. Pre-delivery Hb should be maximised, and red cell loss should be minimised. This may involve the aggressive use of haematinics, rHuEPO, and drugs to decrease operative blood loss.

4. Senior staff with technical expertise should be involved, and consideration should be given to the controversial techniques of acute normovolaemic haemodilution for elective high-risk surgery, and cell salvage with leucocyte depletion filtration for both elective and emergency procedures involving actual or expected massive haemorrhage.

Further reading

Association of Anaesthetists. *Management of Anaesthesia for Jehovah's Witnesses.* Association of Anaesthetists of Great Britain and Ireland. Alresford Press, 1999.

Braga J, Marques R, Branco A, *et al.* Maternal and perinatal implications of the use of human recombinant erythropoietin. *Acta Obstetrica Gynaecologica Scandinavica* 1996; **75**: 449–53.

British Committee for Standards in Haematology Blood Tranfusion Task Force. Guideline for autologous transfusion. II Perioperative haemodilution and cell salvage. *British Journal of Anaesthesia* 1997; **78**: 768–71.

Cane RD. Hb: how much is enough? *Critical Care Medicine* 1990; **18**: 1046–7.

Catling SJ, Williams S, Fielding A. Cell salvage in obstetrics: an evaluation of cell salvage combined with leucocyte depletion filtration to remove amniotic fluid from operative blood loss at caesarean section. *International Journal of Obstetric Anesthesia* 1999; **8**: 79–84.

Erslev AJ. Erythropoeitin. *New England Journal of Medicine* 1991; **324**: 1339–44.

Gould SA, Rosen Al, Lakshman R, *et al.* Fluosol – DA as a red cell substitute in acute anaemia. *New England Journal of Medicine* 1986; **314**: 1653–6.

Howell PJ, Bamber PA. Severe acute anaemia in a Jehovah's Witness. *Anaesthesia* 1987; **42**: 44–8.

Kitchens CS. Are transfusions overrated? Surgical outcome of Jehovah's Witnesses. *American Journal of Medicine* 1993; **94**: 117–19.

Klein HG. The prospects for red cell substitutes. *New England Journal of Medicine* 2000; **342**: 1666–8.

McLoughlin PL, Cope TM, Harrison JC. Hyperbaric oxygen therapy in the management of severe acute anaemia in a Jehovah's Witness. *Anaesthesia* 1999; **54**: 891–4.

Oei SG, Wingen CBM, Kerkkamp HEM. Cell salvage: how safe in obstetrics? (Letter). *International Journal of Obstetric Anesthesia* 2000; **9**: 143.

Report of the Confidential Enquiries into Maternal Deaths in the United Kingdom 1991–1993. Department of Health, Welsh Office, Scottish Office Home and Health Department, Department of Health and Social Services Northern Ireland. HMSO, London, 1996.

Vora M, Gruslin A. Erythropoietin in obstetrics. *Obstetrical and Gynecological Survey* 1998; **53**: 500–8.

Waters JH, Biscotti MD, Potter PS, Phillipson E. Amniotic fluid removal during cell salvage in the cesarian section patient. *Anesthesiology* 2000; **92**: 1531–6.

Weiskopf RB. Erythrocyte salvage during cesarian section. *Anesthesiology* 2000; **92**: 1519–22.

10

A MOTHER WITH KLIPPEL–FEIL SYNDROME: THE PROBLEMS OF KYPHOSCOLIOSIS AND A POTENTIALLY DIFFICULT INTUBATION

A. Bagwell and R. Collis

CASE HISTORY

A 27-year-old woman with well-documented Klippel–Feil syndrome was referred to the obstetric anaesthetic clinic at 30 weeks gestation with a plan for an elective Caesarean section at 36 weeks gestation. The early date for her delivery was a result of steadily deteriorating respiratory function and the need for experienced medical staff to be present for her delivery.

As a child, she had undergone bone grafting and spinal fusion from the mid-cervical to the lower thoracic region in an attempt to arrest a progressive kyphoscoliosis. This was followed by a partial scapulectomy on the left to correct a Sprengels shoulder deformity. As a teenager, she had also been treated for a pulmonary embolus with warfarin, and because of her history of thrombosis, had been started on celaxane when she became pregnant. She had also suffered from recurrent chest infections. She had a peripheral neuropathy, which affected her lower limbs and had required the amputation of several of her toes. This was associated with closed spina bifida of the lumbar vertebra. In order to combat this problem, the neurosurgeons had inserted a spinal cord stimulator, which had been unsuccessful in preventing further deterioration, but at this time an experienced anaesthetist had noted on the anaesthetic chart that she was a 'tricky' intubation (Grade 2b) with the arytenoids only just visible.

Upon direct questioning, our patient admitted extreme shortness of breath upon exertion with an exercise tolerance approaching 50 yards combined with a two-pillow orthopnoea. Physical examination revealed a slim patient with a gross deformity of both spine and chest, which was worse on the left, with a scar running from the upper to lower thoracic spine (Figure 10.1). Auscultation of both the cardiovascular and respiratory systems was unremarkable.

Radiological review of an assortment of X-rays that had been performed several years prior to her pregnancy showed a severe kyphoscoliosis, spina bifida from L3 to sacrum, hemivertebrae in the mid-thoracic spine and multiple ribs originating from one vertebrae (Figure 10.2). A magnetic resonance image (MRI) that was 10 years old, showed that the spinal cord terminated at L3, the absence of an epidural space in association with her spina bifida from L3 downwards and a large dural sac below this level.

Pre-pregnancy respiratory function tests (from an admission 2 years previously) are shown in Table 10.1.

A long discussion in the obstetric anaesthetic clinic resulted in a decision to attempt a regional technique for her Caesarean section, despite the possible difficulties. A combined spinal–epidural (CSE) was felt to be the most appropriate regional technique in this situation, but because of her spina bifida and low termination of the conus, it was not possible to use a needle-through-needle technique. An epidural had to be sited above the termination of the conus and a spinal injection was planned to be injected as low as possible through the spina bifida. Also, in view of the history of difficulties during a previous intubation, as the patient was now 10 kg heavier than on the previous occasion and assessment of her airway predicted a difficult intubation due to her short neck with very little atlanto-occipital movement, fibre-optic intubation equipment was immediately available.

On arriving at the anaesthetic room, non-invasive monitoring was commenced. A 14G intravenous cannula was sited and a fluid preload was started using Hartmann's solution 1000 ml. The patient was then placed in the sitting position with a subjective assessment of a straight spine being obtained. A small dose of lidocaine was then infiltrated over the L2/3 interspace and a 16G-Tuohy needle was inserted using an aseptic technique. Loss of resistance to saline was found at 4 cm and the epidural catheter was inserted without difficulty, with 4 cm remaining in the epidural space. Asepsis was maintained and further lidocaine was infiltrated at the L4/5 interspace. A 20G introducer was positioned and a 25G-Whitacre spinal needle inserted. Clear cerebrospinal fluid (CSF) was obtained at first pass and 2 ml of heavy bupivacaine 0.5% injected together with 20 μg of fentanyl and 100 μg of morphine intrathecally. The patient was then placed in the left lateral position with supplementary oxygen while the block was established. During this time cardiotocograph (CTG) monitoring was commenced.

Despite the very easy injection of the spinal bupivacaine, there was very limited spread of the subarachnoid block, which was not improved by saline injection through the epidural catheter. Three 5 ml boluses of 0.5% bupivacaine epidurally produced a much improved block, but there was limited spread to T6 on the left side. We assumed this to be caused by abnormalities within the epidural space caused by her previous stabilisation surgery to her thoracic curvature.

The initial incision passed without incident, but three boluses of 25 μg of intravenous fentanyl were required for supplemental analgesia intra-operatively. The procedure itself was uncomplicated and a healthy baby girl weighing 2150 g was delivered with Apgar scores of 9 at 1 min and 10 at 5 min. No obvious physical abnormality or subsequent radiological evidence of abnormalities was detected.

Post-operative recovery was unremarkable and excellent analgesia was provided by the intrathecal opioids and rectal diclofenac over the first 24 h. She did require intramuscular (IM) morphine on a number of occasions over the following 3 days. Following regression of the block, no new neurological problems were found.

Both mother and baby were discharged 9 days post-operatively, fit and well.

DESCRIPTION OF THE PROBLEM

1. Servere kyphoscoliosis with or without previous corrective or stabilisation surgery can cause technical difficulties when siting a regional block.

2. If surgery is very extensive, general anaesthesia may be the only option for Caesarean section.

3. Spinal and epidural anaesthesia may be patchy or unpredictable either because of the abnormal curvature of the spine or because of abnormalities within the epidural space.

4. Kyphoscoliosis can be associated with marked cardiac and respiratory impairment if severe.

5. Kyphoscoliosis is associated with other major abnormalities of the spinal column, such as spina bifida.

6. Kyphoscoliosis is associated with a number of different congenital problems, Klippel–Feil syndrome being only one.

7. Difficult intubation can be predicted with some syndromes, such as Klippel–Feil syndrome.

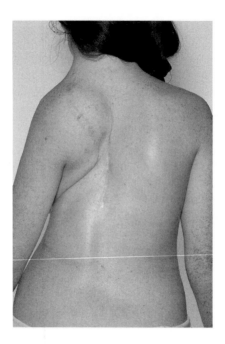

Figure 10.1

PATHOPHYSIOLOGY

In our case, the patient had severe kyphoscoliosis in association with Klippel–Feil syndrome. The pathophysiology of the syndrome had to be considered in association with the problems of spinal anatomy as well as respiratory compromise.

Limited respiratory function will cause difficulties as the increased respiratory demands of pregnancy cannot be met easily. The mother will not be able to meet an increase in minute ventilation of up to 50% with increased tidal volumes, and she will become progressively dyspnoeic. As the pregnancy encroaches on her diaphragm she will find it difficult to cough effectively and is, therefore, more likely to develop chest infections. It is also likely that due to the fore-shortening of the vertebral column, the pregnancy may be encroaching into the chest by the mid-second trimester.

Bony anomalies

Epidural anaesthesia may be technically difficult to perform because of the significant anatomical abnormalities, such as thoracic kyphoscoliosis, making bony landmarks difficult to identify. Fusion of vertebrae and a narrowed epidural space may make identification of the extradural space more difficult and increases the risk of a dural puncture. There may also be subsequent difficulty in inserting the epidural catheter to a sufficient depth. As with all pregnant patients, the epidural

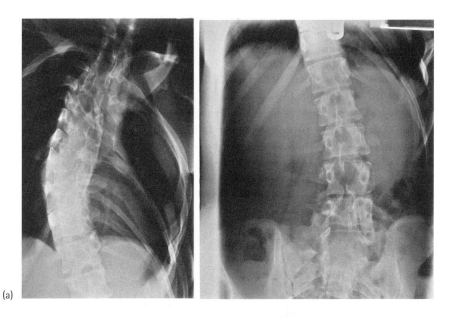

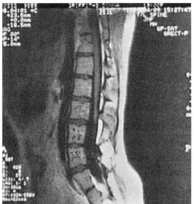

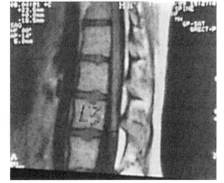

(a)

(b)

Figure 10.2

Table 10.1

	Predicted	Measured	Percentage
VC (l)	3.2	0.88	23
FVC (l)	3.4	0.83	23
FEV1 (l)	3.4	0.85	27
PEF (l/min)	450	132	30

veins are also more engorged than usual, thus increasing the risk of intravascular catheter insertion. The consequent injection of the local anaesthetic mixture may also be unpredictable and inadequate.

Our patient also had closed spina bifida. There were no anomalies noted on her skin covering the lumbar spine but she was aware of the problem and review of her X-rays confirmed this. With any grade of spina bifida, there can be abnormal tethering of the spinal cord resulting in an abnormally low termination of the conus. Only detailed X-rays and scans can determine where regional anaesthesia can safely be performed.

Due to the bony abnormalities of the cervical vertebra, patients with Klippel–Feil syndrome can be very difficult to intubate. Type I Klippel–Feil is an extensive abnormality whereby elements of both cervical and thoracic vertebrae are incorporated in a single fused block. In type II Klipple–Feil, failure of complete segmentation occurs at one or two cervical interspaces and is associated with hemivertebrae and occipito-atlantal fusion. Type III Klipple–Feil includes type I or II deformities with co-existing segmentation defects in the thoracic and lumbar spines. Inheritance of the syndrome includes both autosomal dominant and recessive mechanisms, which are yet to be fully elucidated.

MANAGEMENT OPTIONS AND DISCUSSION

Regional anaesthesia

All regional techniques may be technically demanding and should be performed by the most experienced operator available. A single spinal injection may be the best option, avoiding metal fixators and preventing accidental dural puncture with a Tuohy needle, because of scarring in the epidural space. The problem is that there is almost certainly an increased failure rate because of unpredictable spread of the local anaesthetic in the CSF, due to either the abnormal curvature or as in our case other anomalies such as spina bifida.

Epidurals can be sited away from surgical scars and spina bifida but they may work very unpredictably. The epidural space will be distorted and scarred leading to uneven distribution of local anaesthetic. Epidurals may be very disappointing under these circumstances but can be worth trying for labour analgesia if the mother is agreeable.

A CSE may offer the greatest flexibility and best quality of block when compared to the two discrete procedures. The choice the operator faces is whether to employ a single or dual space technique to achieve the required block. In our patient there was no level where the epidural space existed without risking damage to the conus behind; therefore, it was mandatory in our case to use a dual space technique. However, there may be only a single suitable entry point for needle insertion, making a needle-through-needle approach the better option.

By using a CSE with a low–dose spinal component, it would be theoretically possible to tailor the block height exactly to the individual requirement, without compromising respiratory function. This technique is also safer for those patients who have had a failed intubation. Many patients have a strong preference to be awake for the delivery and by combining local anaesthetic in the subarachnoid and epidural space it may reduce the shortcomings of the individual injections, but a general anaesthetic may still need to be employed.

Another technique that has been described is that of an intrathecal catheter. This has been utilised with both single shot and as an incremental spinal technique via a microspinal catheter. The use of a microspinal catheter permits the controlled onset of spinal anaesthesia without sudden circulatory changes and furthermore the chance of an excessively high block in these unpredictable cases. The smallest catheters have been withdrawn, because of an association with cauda equina syndrome, but larger catheters can still be used, although due to the size of the introducer needle they may be associated with an unacceptable rate of postdural puncture headache. Experience in the UK is limited, however, making the technique more theoretically advantageous.

General anaesthesia

The management of a patient undergoing Caesarean section who has Klippel–Feil syndrome is fraught with difficulties relating to both difficult intubation, possible acid aspiration and difficulty in extubation in those patients with respiratory compromise. Cardiorespiratory function may be impaired by several factors specific to Klippel–Feil syndrome with thoracic kyphoscoliosis, upper airway obstruction, rib deformities and recurrent chest infections being common.

In view of the likely difficulty in tracheal intubation, it is essential that the airway is secured before induction of general anaesthesia. In elective surgical cases, there is ample time to consider a number of different approaches. Patients with spondylosis or hypermobility are at risk of spinal cord injury during medical procedures, such as laryngoscopy, tracheal intubation and operative positioning. Indeed, care of the occipito-cervical junction often requires the provision of rigid support for the patient's head, neck and shoulders before loss of muscle tone. It has been suggested that awake nasal fibre-optic assessment of the airway under local analgesia should be undertaken as an outpatient before admitting the patient. This would give useful information concerning the anatomy, condition of nerves, pharynx and the laryngeal inlet. Review articles have suggested that the flexible fibrescope should be used much more as a routine part of the perioperative management of patients, especially those suspected of having upper or lower airway pathology or distorted anatomy from other causes.

The best conditions for fibre-optic intubation are found in an awake patient, since they can assist in clearing their own secretions, phonating or panting. In the obstetric patient the additional risk of regurgitation makes the awake technique the only one acceptable. Fibre-optic intubation is, therefore, not suitable if intubation has failed in the obstetric situation but is best carried out in the elective, anticipated difficult intubation setting. The nasal route is preferred since the tongue is less likely to interfere, and the patient cannot interrupt the procedure by biting down. Other problems include difficulty in performing transtracheal injections and superior laryngeal nerve blocks due to the patients being unable to extend their neck.

Awake intubation technique

Before employing an awake fibre-optic intubation, the technique must be adequately explained to the patient. This is best done away from the anaesthetic room where a more relaxed and comprehensive discussion can take place.

The technique we currently use is as follows: xylometazolin is sprayed into the nose initially. The nose is then anaesthetised with cotton tipped buds soaked in 4% lidocaine (0.5 ml to each nostril). The throat and pharynx is anaesthetised with 10% lidocaine spray ($\times 12 = 120$ mg) through the mouth. The larynx is then anaesthetised with two lots of 2 ml of 2% lidocaine squirted down an epidural catheter inserted through the suction port of the fibrescope. Mild sedation for the procedure is provided with fentanyl and midazolam. A well lubricated size 6.0 reinforced Mallinkrodt cuffed tracheal tube is then inserted into the trachea. Once placement is confirmed, the patient is anaesthetised.

Prior to extubation, any reduction in neuromuscular transmission must be reversed in order to maximise the patient's respiratory function. Added to this, sleep induced ventilatory dysfunction may occur in patients with structural central nervous system lesions. The patient should be extubated awake in the left lateral position. However, provision should be made for an intensive care bed to be available if there is any significant respiratory compromise in the post-operative period. These patients should be nursed in a high-dependency environment postoperatively, irrespective of the anaesthetic technique employed.

General points

Policy regarding patients with Klippel–Feil syndrome should be to ensure an elective procedure with experienced personnel from all relevant specialities. There is great benefit from careful clinical review and radiological assessment. An anaesthetic obstetric assessment clinic offers a point of referral for obstetric staff and this allows ideas for analgesia and anaesthesia to be exchanged between both patient and anaesthetist in a relaxed and controlled environment.

KEY LEARNING POINTS

1. Klippel–Feil syndrome is a multisystem disorder with primarily skeletal abnormalities.

2. General anaesthesia can be complicated by difficult intubation and poor respiratory function.

3. Regional anaesthesia can be technically difficult but may offer the most effective way of providing anaesthesia.

4. Careful pre-operative history and examination should be made of all patients with Klippel–Feil syndrome and appropriate investigations ordered.

5. All patients with significant kyphoscoliosis with or without a previous history of surgery will benefit from a thorough review in an obstetric anaesthetic clinic.

Further reading

Collier CB. *An Atlas of Epidurograms: Epidural Blocks Investigated*. Martin Punitz, London, 1998, Chapter 7.

Daum R, Jones D. Fibreoptic intubation in Klippel–Feil syndrome. *Anaesthesia* 1998; **43**: 18–21.

Dresner M, Maclean A. Anaesthesia for Caesarean section in a patient with Klippel–Feil syndrome. The use of a microspinal catheter. *Anaesthesia* 1995; **50**: 807–9.

Naguib M, Farag H, Ibrahim A. Anaesthetic considerations in Klippel–Feil syndrome. *Canadian Anaesthetists Society Journal* 1986; **33**: 66–70.

11

THE OBSTETRIC PATIENT WITH LATEX ALLERGY

J.C. Hughes

CASE HISTORY

A 32-year-old female, gravida 2, para 1, presented for elective lower segment Caesarean section. Her first child was born by emergency Caesarean section under spinal anaesthesia. During this procedure, she developed an anaphylactic reaction and was successfully resuscitated with boluses of epinephrine. Blood taken for mast cell tryptase levels 1 h after the reaction confirmed that histamine release had taken place. Subsequent serologic examination for latex-specific IgE antibodies (RAST) and skin tests confirmed the diagnosis of allergy to latex. Following this episode, she was forced to leave her job as an intensive care nurse because her employers were unable to guarantee a latex-free environment.

This pregnancy had been uneventful, and she was now 39 weeks gestation. There was a history of asthma, which was probably related to exposure to airborne latex allergens. Close questioning also revealed previous episodes of lip swelling after inflation of a balloon, and also an allergy to kiwi fruit.

This lady was identified to anaesthetic staff early on in pregnancy as a case of latex allergy and after discussion with the anaesthetist, patient and midwifery staff, a plan was formulated to deal with the elective Caesarean section, which the patient had requested. It was considered preferable to perform an elective rather than a rushed emergency Caesarean section in the middle of the night after an unsuccessful trial of labour. The plan was formulated after reference to the hospital latex allergy protocol, and was disseminated to all staff that might come into contact with the patient.

Prior to surgery, the Central Sterile Services Department (CSSD) was requested to process two standard Caesarean section surgical trays using either no gloves, or latex-free gloves, prior to sterilisation by autoclave. They were also required to remove all latex items from the tray, including elastic bands, suction tubing, etc. Both trays were made available for the operation. On the evening prior to surgery, the operating theatre to be used was meticulously cleaned by cleaning personnel wearing latex-free gloves, having thoroughly washed their hands prior to donning gloves. All non-essential equipment and products containing latex were removed from the theatre and essential equipment cleaned. The theatre doors were marked with a 'no-entry, latex-free area' sign, and any emergency surgery during the night was carried out in another theatre.

On the morning of surgery, the theatre was again cleaned at 6 a.m. and left to rest until 9 a.m. Only designated staffs wearing clean theatre clothes were allowed entry to the theatre and they were required to wash their hands prior to donning latex-free gloves.

The patient received a standard premedication consisting of oral ranitidine 150 mg the night before and on the morning of surgery, and sodium citrate 30 ml immediately prior to anaesthesia. All anaesthetic and surgical equipment was checked to ensure that it was latex free. Items for which the latex-free status was unknown were either not used, or their status was confirmed with the manufacturer. This included the operating table mattress, monitoring equipment including blood pressure cuff, intravenous cannulae, syringes, spinal needles, filter needles, breathing system and ventilator bellows, face-masks (including Hudson mask), tracheal tubes, urinary catheter, surgical equipment and all gloves. Antibiotics were drawn up after first removing the rubber stopper from the ampoule. Resuscitation drugs and equipment were available in case a reaction should occur despite all precautions.

In the event, the patient had an uncomplicated Caesarean section under spinal anaesthesia and was transferred back to the post-natal ward with instructions to continue avoidance of latex, including the use of latex-free gloves by domestic staff handing out food. She made an unremarkable recovery and now wears a 'Medic-Alert' bracelet warning future carers about her latex allergy.

DEFINITION OF THE PROBLEM

Since its initial recognition in 1979, latex allergy has become increasingly recognised as a problem for some surgical patients, particularly in the USA, but also now in the UK and Europe. The anaesthetist may be faced with a patient who is known to be allergic to latex and will require special precautions. More worryingly, latex allergy may present intra-operatively as an anaphylactic reaction.

PATHOPHYSIOLOGY

Latex is a natural product from the rubber tree *Hevea brazilienses* and latex products have been used in the medical field since the late 19th century. Three types of reaction have been described:

1. Local skin irritation.

2. Type IV (delayed) hypersensitivity reaction, which tends to cause eczematous contact dermatitis.

3. Type I (anaphylactic) reaction mediated via IgE, which tends to cause a full blown anaphylactic reaction as a result of mediator release.

Latex allergy is more common in certain groups of patients (see Table 11.1). There also appears to be a cross reactivity with certain fruits such as bananas, kiwi fruit, chestnut and avocado. There is a worrying incidence of latex allergy in healthcare workers, and 17% of healthcare workers are skin prick positive, varying from 38% in dental personnel compared to 9% of physicians. The incidence in the general population is about 1%, but this rises to as much as 60% in those with spina bifida.

MANAGEMENT OPTIONS AND DISCUSSION

Investigation of suspected cases

It has been suggested that all patients presenting for operation should be questioned about latex allergy, and those who give a positive history, or those falling into one of the high-risk groups, should be offered testing for latex allergy. This may include serologic evaluation for the presence of latex-specific IgE (RAST test) and/or skin prick tests. Patients with a strong history of latex allergy should be managed in a latex-free environment, even if immunological tests are negative. A positive history combined with raised total serum IgE has 78% sensitivity and 91%

Table 11.1 – Patients considered at high-risk of latex allergy.

Patients with a history of atopy
Occupational exposure to rubber products
Healthcare workers
Patients with disorders such as spina bifida
Patients undergoing repetitive urinary instrumentation
Patients undergoing repeated operations
Females appear to be more susceptible than males
History of anaphylaxis of uncertain aetiology, especially if associated
 with previous surgery, hospitalisations or dental visits

specificity in predicting those at risk. Up to a third of atopic subjects frequently exposed to latex will become sensitive.

In the obstetric setting, patients may present with a history of latex allergy or fall into one of the high-risk groups, but they may also present *de novo* with an allergic reaction. It is important to recognise that a patient does not have to have an operation to have a reaction, but may be exposed to latex during catheterisation or vaginal examination, or by inhaling airborne latex, which is often present in the hospital environment. For this reason, it is vital that local protocols exist for the management of these patients, whether it is to treat a reaction once it has occurred or to prevent one occurring in a patient known to be susceptible.

Protocols for managing latex allergy

A number of protocols exist, but whichever is chosen, it should be adapted to fit local circumstances and then disseminated widely to those likely to be involved in the care of a patient with latex allergy. They should also be updated regularly. All protocols stress the importance of identifying those at risk and then avoiding exposure to latex, at all stages during the healthcare process. This means that all healthcare workers involved in the care of such patients are aware of the problems and how to manage them. Latex avoidance in at-risk patients may be exemplary during surgery, but vigilance needs to be continued throughout the hospital stay. When the patient returns to the ward, they should ideally be placed in a 'clean' side room. Something as innocuous as preparation of the patient's food using latex gloves may set off a reaction.

The anaesthetist should be aware of the 'latex status' of all equipment in use (see Table 11.2). Manufacturers are becoming increasingly aware of this problem, and many devices now do not contain latex. Some medications are only presented in vials with rubber stoppers. These should be removed from the vial before drawing up the drug. The best way to avoid a problem is to routinely use latex-free products. If this is not possible a 'latex-free cart' can be made up containing equipment to be used on a patient with latex allergy. An extensive website lists the latex status of

Table 11.2 – Equipment potentially containing latex.

Airways	ECG electrode pads
Masks	Intravenous bags and giving sets
Rebreathing bags	Medication vials
Breathing circuit tubing	Stethoscope tubing
Band-aids and adhesive tape	Suction catheters
Blood pressure cuffs	Tourniquets
Syringes	Mattresses
Urinary catheters	Spinal and epidural packs

many products used in theatre and anaesthesia (http://www.immune.com/rubber/UKDatabase.html). Recent evidence suggests that bacterial and viral filters may protect the patient from airborne latex particles in the breathing system.

Premedication

The premedication of patients with latex allergy is controversial. Some people suggest giving steroids, and histamine (H_1 and H_2) receptor antagonists to attenuate any allergic response should this occur, but others suggest this should be avoided as it may mask the early signs of anaphylaxis. Whichever approach is taken does not reduce the requirements for strict avoidance of exposure of the patient to latex.

KEY LEARNING POINTS

1. Latex allergy is becoming more common, though certain risk groups can be identified.

2. All healthcare workers should be aware of the problem, how to treat it, and how to avoid it.

3. All areas providing healthcare should have a protocol for managing a patient suspected of being allergic to latex.

4. Patients may present with an anaphylactic reaction and this should be presumed to be due to latex until proven otherwise, particularly if it presents intra-operatively.

Further reading

American Association of Nurse Anaesthetists. Latex allergy protocol. *Journal of the American Association of Nurse Anaesthetists* 1993; **61**: 223–4.

Association of Anaesthetists. *Suspected Anaphylactic Reactions Associated with Anaesthesia 2 (Revised Edition)*. The Association of Anaesthetists of Great Britain and Ireland, 1995.

Barbara J, Chabane MH, Leynadier F, Girard F. Retention of airborne latex particles by a bacterial and viral filter used in anaesthesia. *Anaesthesia* 2001; **56**: 231–4.

Dakin MJ, Yentis SM. Latex allergy: a strategy for management. *Anaesthesia* 1998; **53**: 774–81.

Kelly KJ, Pearson ML, Kurup VP, *et al.* A cluster of anaphylactic reactions in children with spina bifida during general anesthesia: epidemiologic features, risk factors, and latex hypersensitivity. *Journal of Allergy and Clinical Immunology* 1994; **94**: 53–61.

McKinnon RP. Allergic reactions during anaesthesia. *Current Opinion in Anesthesiology* 1996; **9**: 267–70.

Moneret-Vautrin D-A, Beaudouin E, Widmer S, *et al.* Prospective study of risk factors in natural rubber latex hypersensitivity. *Journal of Allergy and Clinical Immunology* 1993; **92**: 668–77.

Nutter AF. Contact urticaria to rubber. *British Journal of Dermatology* 1979; **101**: 597–8. http://www.jr2.ox.ac.uk/Bandolier/bandopubs/NHSSlatex.html

Pollard RJ, Layon AJ. Latex allergy in the operating room: case report and a brief review of the literature. *Journal of Clinical Anesthesia* 1996; **8**: 161–7.

Santos R, Hernandez-Ayup S, Galache P, Morales FG, Batiza VA, Montoya D. Severe latex allergy after a vaginal examination during labor: a case report. *American Journal of Obstetric Gynecology* 1997; **177**: 1543–4.

Silverman HI. Rubber anaphylaxis. *New England Journal of Medicine* 1989; **320**: 1126–30.

Task force on allergic reactions to latex. *Journal of Allergy and Clinical Immunology* 1993; **92**: 16–18.

Understanding Latex in the Perioperative Setting. National Association of Theatre Nurses (UK), 2000.

Weiss ME, Hirshman CA. Latex allergy. Editorial. *Canadian Journal of Anaesthesia* 1992; **39**: 528–32.

Yassin MS, Lierl MB, Fischer TJ, O'Brien K, Cross J, Steinmetz C. Latex allergy in hospital employees. *Annals of Allergy* 1994; **72**: 245–9.

12

A LEGAL ASPECT OF OBSTETRIC ANAESTHESIA: *BOLAM* REDEFINED

C.P.H. Heneghan

CASE HISTORY

The patient was a 36-year-old management consultant at term with her first child, listed for elective Caesarean section for maternal request. Following an explanation of the risk of headache, feeling some discomfort during the operative procedure, weakness for 2–4 h, and of slight risk of nerve damage, she consented to a spinal anaesthetic.

At 13.30 h, she was positioned in the left lateral position, 'skin-prepped', draped and the skin anaesthetised by a consultant anaesthetist, who was fully scrubbed and gloved and in a theatre hat. A 24 G Sprotte was introduced at L3/4 in the midline. Dural puncture with good cerebrospinal fluid (CSF) flow-back was easily achieved, and 2.5 ml heavy bupivacaine 0.5% + 0.1 mg preservative-free morphine were injected, and she was turned into the supine tilt position. A block from T5-caudal bilaterally was achieved, testing with a sharp sterile point, and surgery proceeded uneventfully with the delivery of a live male infant weighing 3.2 kg. Postoperatively, she was nursed in labour ward for 2 h and then returned to the ward, pain free. She received two co-proxamol tablets 4 hourly three times, and the following morning was well and out of bed. Later that day, she began to complain of a headache, and was advised by the midwifery staff to lie down and was given more co-proxamol.

At 17.00 h, an anaesthetist was asked to review her headache as it was felt that it may be connected with her spinal anaesthetic. She was unable to attend immediately and 2 h later, the anaesthetist was called again. She eventually came to the antenatal ward at 20.00 h, 1 h after that. The patient still had a severe headache, and cried out and rolled away when the light was turned on in her room. On examination, she had a stiff neck and seemed a little confused as she repeatedly asked if her baby was alright, and where her husband was, though they had both been in the room with her until just before the anaesthetist arrived. The midwife pointed out that the patient's temperature was 39°C, and she had been having rigours.

The anaesthetist diagnosed a spinal headache, and prescribed diclofenac suppositories to supplement the co-proxamol, which she thought may be causing dysphoria or hallucinations. To be on the safe side, she called the consultant who performed the spinal, who accepted the assessment, though suggested perhaps a medical opinion in view of the patient's temperature, as she may be developing a postoperative pneumonia. The anaesthetist referred the patient to the on-call junior physician, who arrived to review her at 24.00 h. He was informed by the midwifery staff, that the patient had settled after the diclofenac, but when he went into her room, he found she was unrousable, with a Glasgow Coma Score of three, stertorous breathing and a temperature of 41°C. She was immediately admitted to intensive care, intubated and ventilated. She had a lumbar puncture that revealed turbid purulent CSF, which subsequently grew a salivary streptococcus, also found in the blood culture and subsequently in the consultant anaesthetist's nasal swab. Antibiotic treatment was started, she woke up over the next 2 days and was weaned off the ventilator on the morning of the fourth postoperative day. Her subsequent recovery was steady, though she had clearly sustained significant brain damage, and remained severely disabled, needing full-time nursing care, with no prospect of ever returning to work. She sued, and damages for pain suffering and loss of amenity are estimated at £50,000, with loss of earnings based on salary and bonuses of £500,000 pa totalled to £7.5 million, and nursing and other support costs totalled to £1.8 million. Total damages and costs are liable to exceed £10 million.

SETTING OUT THE LEGAL BASIS OF THE CASE

1. The standard of care in medical cases was set out by McNair J in Bolam [1] in 1957. He made it clear that the standard was that of a doctor practising in that field, and that if the standard actually adopted would be accepted by a responsible body of practitioners in the field, even if that body was a minority, that standard was not negligent.

2. It did not matter whether the practice made sense to the court, nor whether by the time the court considered the case, perhaps many years later, the practice had been clearly shown to be wrong.

3. It only mattered that at the time, responsible practitioners thought it was OK.

4. This standard recognised that there are developments in medicine, and that there may be differences of opinion about the efficacy and/or safety of innovations. It recognises that medicine is an inexact science, and that a court should not seek to interpret the science, nor try to decide retrospectively the correctness of a respectable opinion. In this respect, the court accepted the medical view of negligence, and doctors have generally been comfortable with the *Bolam* test.

5. Lawyers, especially those representing Complainants, have not been so comfortable, seeing the situation as one where one doctor is asked whether another has been negligent, and (unsurprisingly, the lawyers think) says 'no'. While one may wonder what this reveals about lawyers' thinking, one can see the force of the argument, especially in the light of the journalistic clichés about doctors closing ranks.

6. Over the decades since 1957, the courts have witnessed a war of attrition against *Bolam* reminiscent of renaissance explorers' search for the Northwest Passage (to China, via a route north of the American continent). Numerous different routes have been explored, eventually a workable route round *Bolam* at last being found. I have used a hypothetical amalgam of cases to illustrate the point (comment on a real case might have untoward legal consequences).

EXPERT OPINIONS

Expert opinions can be summarised as follows:

Complainant's expert advises that there can be no criticism of the decision to offer spinal anaesthesia, nor of the technique, except that not to wear a mask is falling below the proper standard. Postoperative management was of an acceptable standard until the delay in attendance by the anaesthetist; not coming until 3 h after being called; the failure to diagnose or consider meningitis in spite of the failure to respond to lying flat, the very high temperature with confusion and photophobia; the diagnosis of spinal headache; the failure to start antibiotics at that point; the failure of midwifery staff to monitor properly or at all between 20.00 and 24.00 h; the failure of the physician to attend for 4 h after being called. Treatment thereafter was of high standard, but by then the damage was done.

Defendants' experts agreed that the technique was proper, disagreed that it was falling below the proper standard to fail to wear a mask as a responsible minority of practitioners still regarded it as acceptable to perform spinals or epidurals unmasked; agreed that the standard of care was acceptable until the point where the anaesthetist was first called, felt the delay in attending was justifiable as the anaesthetist was performing two Caesarean section anaesthetics and an epidural between 17.00 and 19.45 h, and while she did eat a sandwich before seeing the patient, this delay of 15 min would not have changed the eventual outcome. He accepted that meningitis was within the differential diagnosis at this point, but rejected the suggestion that it was falling below the proper standard to fail to diagnosis or treat it, as this is very uncommon and unlikely. (He also rejected the suggestion that the anaesthetist had failed to consider the diagnosis, as the anaesthetist said she did think of it, though did not write it down or act on it!) The delay by the physician, he said, was justifiable as he had had 17 admissions between 17.30 and 23.15 h, and it was commendable, especially since it was unclear from the referral that there was a serious problem, that he saw the patient as soon as he did. Treatment thereafter was agreed to be of high quality.

After a joint meeting of experts, it was agreed that the points at issue were:

1. Was it acceptable not to wear a mask during spinal anaesthesia?

2. Was it acceptable not to diagnose meningitis at the anaesthetist's 20.00 h visit, or at least to prescribe antibiotics in view of the high temperature?

Complainant's expert advised the Complainant's lawyers that it would probably not be possible to sustain the allegation of negligence as to the failure to diagnose meningitis, as the anaesthetist is not a specialist in that field. The only point at issue was thus whether it was negligent to fail to wear a mask, as it was accepted by both sides that this failure, if negligent, had probably caused or materially contributed to the patient's acquiring meningitis.

Defendant's expert can show that while there is a vocal and convincing body of opinion, which supports wearing of masks, there is also evidence that it makes no difference, and that the incidence of meningitis following spinals is no different to the sporadic incidence in a similar group of patients. Indeed, there is evidence that even when masks are worn, meningitis may still follow. Accordingly, the practice of not wearing a mask was an acceptable minority practice.

Complainant's expert could show that wearing of masks could completely prevent bacterial dispersal resultant on talking [2], and that while there were reported cases in which masks had been worn and meningitis still developed [3,4], and it could be argued that the incidence of bacterial meningitis after spinal anaesthesia is no greater than in the population as a whole [5], nevertheless the risk was very substantially reduced by wearing a mask, and the failure to do so probably caused or materially contributed to the development of meningitis. Until recently, the matter would probably have rested there, the responsible minority view winning the day. However, recent developments change that.

LEGAL ANALYSIS

The law set out in *Bolam* was reasonably clear: if a responsible minority of practitioners supported a course of action, it was not negligent. Other words have been used interchangeably with responsible, such as respectable or reputable, but the sense was the same: if some good doctors did this, it was OK. What makes the body responsible had been litigated, and in a recent case [6] it is interesting to observe that publication of a series of cases in the BJA was by itself not sufficient to make a very unusual course of action responsible, though a properly designed scientific study might have been. Being in a minority of one did not necessarily debar responsibleness, nor did being in a nascent speciality [7].

In a complex case involving a number of points (*Bolitho* [8]), a case of similar antiquity to *Bolam* was unearthed and referred to the court (*Hucks v Cole* [9]). In this case, only reported contemporaneously with *Bolitho*, a patient developed septic spots in the post-partum period. She was treated with an antibiotic blind, and got better. Microbiology of the septic spots revealed bacteria insensitive to the antibiotic prescribed, though sensitive to another. The general practitioner (GP) managing the case did not prescribe the second antibiotic, reasoning that the patient was well and it was unnecessary. Subsequently, the patient became seriously ill with septic shock and although she did eventually recover, she sued and won! In spite of the fact that a range of the most eminent experts in the land (including Dame Josephine Barnes) gave evidence that they would not have given antibiotics in the circumstances, the court decided that it could reject that view and substitute its own. On the basis that it was agreed that had the patient been given the second antibiotic she would not then have developed septic shock, and that it was a simple matter to give the (cheap and ordinary) antibiotic, the court said it was not logical to withold it, and therefore not defensible.

This surprising judgement has been upheld in the House of Lords in *Bolitho* [8], and is now the law. The Lords put a slightly different gloss on it, however, saying that when a court came to assess whether the action of a body of practitioners was responsible, respectable or reputable, it could have recourse to logical analysis. The Lords will always try to produce a judgement which apparently overturns as little as possible of pre-existing law, as it otherwise means having to admit that previous judgements – perhaps some of their own! – were wrong. Thus rather than state that *Bolam*, many time approved in the Lords, was wrong, they say that it merely needs to be interpreted slightly differently, albeit that this interpretation is virtually 180° from previous interpretations. This has resulted in it now frequently being pleaded that the defendant doctor's course of action was negligent because it was not logical.

In the hypothetical case I am discussing, it would be alleged that it was not logical not to wear a mask. While there may be an entirely respectable body of medical opinion which agrees that wearing a mask is unnecessary, nevertheless it is a minor and cheap intervention to put on a mask, it would probably have prevented the untoward outcome, and it is not logical to fail to do so, thus it is negligent to fail to do so. There is thus a serious risk that this case would be won by the Complainant using this argument.

DISCUSSION

This is a hypothetical case. In the circumstances where there are prospects of winning around £10 million for a Complainant, and in the event an enormously enhanced reputation for themselves, there can be little doubt that the lawyers would pursue all possible avenues. Were this particular factual point to be the turning point of a case, I think it highly likely that it would be forcefully argued, and probable that it would succeed. Though some lawyers think *Bolitho* will have little effect on deciding clinical negligence cases, it seems to me that the responsible minority *Bolam* defence will be considerably less applicable than before. How should this cause us to change our practice?

We can no longer rely on the defence that what we do is accepted by a responsible minority. If the alternative proposed is logically superior, or appears so to the court, especially if the logical analysis is relatively simple, there is a serious risk that our practice will be found to be negligent. What can we do?

The problem is predicting what a judge will think is logical and simple. My hypothetical case has not as far as I know been litigated. However, it seems to me to fit (and I have started wearing masks when I do spinals). We may all be able to think of such examples, and might persuade ourselves to change practice accordingly. There is, however, a real risk of defensive medicine developing once again, and many unnecessary precautions being taken just in case a judge thinks them logical. No doubt numerous examples of 'logical' precautions will be condemned as cases are litigated, and many of them will seem as unfair as in *Hucks v Cole*. Unfortunately, it will not be easy to predict what the courts will find logical, and it will not be easy to change our practice to anticipate such a finding. Uncertainty in the law is very undesirable, as we cannot know in advance what the law will be if taken to court. Uncertainty does, however, seem to have been achieved by this dubious judgement. Now, more than ever, it is important to keep one's defence organisation subscription paid up.

Note

I have argued the above on the basis of the failure to wear a mask as the only point of dispute. In reality, of course, in such a case as the above I think it extraordinarily unlikely that the experts would agree that it was not negligent for the anaesthetist to fail to diagnose meningitis at the 20.00 h visit, if only on the same 'logical' basis. I have considered another, more commonplace, possible error, as the failure to treat at 20.00 h is very close to the failure in *Hucks v Cole,* and I do not wish to give the impression that this new departure only applies to antibiotic treatment.

KEY LEARNING POINTS

1. We can no longer rely on the defence that 'what we do is accepted by a responsible minority'.

2. If the alternative proposed is logically superior, or appears so to the court, there is a serious risk that our practice will be found to be negligent.

3. There is therefore a real risk of defensive medicine developing.

4. Unfortunately, it will not be easy to predict what the courts will find logical, and it will not be easy to change our practice to anticipate such a finding.

References

[1] *Bolam v Friern HMC* [1957] 1 WLR 582.

[2] Philips BJ, *et al.* Surgical facemasks are effective in reducing bacterial contamination caused by dispersal from the upper airway. *British Journal of Anaesthesia* 1992; **69**: 407–8.

[3] Newton JA, *et al.* Streptococcus salivarius meningitis after spinal anaesthesia. *Clinical Infectious Disease* 1994; **18**: 840–1.

[4] Laurila JJ, *et al.* Streptococcus salivarius meningitis after spinal anaesthesia. *Anesthesiology* 1998; **89**: 1579–80.

[5] Editorial: Meningitis after spinal anaesthesia. *British Journal of Anaesthesia* 1997; **78**: 635–6.

[6] *Hepworth v Kerr* (QBD) [1995] Med LR 139.

[7] *De Freitas v O'Brien & Connolly* (CA) [1995] Med LR 108.

[8] *Bolitho v City & Hackney HA,* [1998] Lloyd's Rep Med 26. HL.

[9] *Hucks v Cole* [1993] 4 MedLR 393 (CA).

13

MALIGNANT HYPERPYREXIA AND PREGNANCY

A. Carling and S. Jeffs

CASE HISTORY 1

A 27-year-old Caucasian woman presented to the antenatal clinic and was referred for an anaesthetic opinion as she was known to be susceptible to malignant hyperpyrexia (MH). The MH Investigation Unit in Leeds had investigated her as a child because she is part of a known positive family. She had previously undergone an uneventful tonsillectomy when the anaesthetic drugs used were thiopentone, fentanyl, pancuronium, nitrous oxide, atropine and neostigmine.

She was fit and well, was taking no medication except folic acid, had no allergies and was a non-smoker. Examination including airway assessment was unremarkable. As a result, an anaesthetic plan was drawn up following discussion with the patient of the potential risks. She agreed to epidural analgesia for labour and a spinal anaesthetic if surgery was required. The midwifery and surgical staff were made aware that the anaesthetic team should be informed as soon as she was admitted in labour.

She was admitted at term in spontaneous labour and an epidural was inserted within 2 h of admission. A test dose of 3.5 ml bupivacaine 0.5% was administered. A good block was established using 10 mls bupivacaine 0.08% with fentanyl 2.5 μg/ml followed by an infusion at 10 ml/h to maintain analgesia. Eight hours later, she was delivered by Ventouse extraction of a baby boy with Apgar scores 9 and 9 at 1 and 5 min, respectively.

The patient was discharged 2 days later having experienced no problems.

CASE HISTORY 2

The obstetric anaesthetic staff reviewed a 35-year-old woman as her son had been diagnosed with central core muscle disease. This is an autosomal dominant condition that can be associated with MH susceptibility (MHS). Neither she nor her husband had any signs or symptoms but it is possible that either might have a mild form of the condition and thus be MHS.

She had previously undergone several uneventful general anaesthetics. As she was to have an elective Caesarean section, a lumbar subarachnoid block was thought to be the best option. This was duly performed without any problems.

She and other members of her family were subsequently investigated for MHS.

DEFINITION OF THE PROBLEM

MH is an inherited disorder, which can be triggered by some anaesthetic agents. Since the introduction of investigation and treatment of MH, the mortality rate has decreased from 70% in the 1960s to 5% today. Most recent estimates of the population prevalence of the genetic susceptibility are between 1 : 5000 and 1 : 10,000. The incidence of reported MH reactions varies from 1 in 40,000 to 1 in 100,000 anaesthetics. Unrecognised and untreated it has a significant mortality rate. Early referral of MHS parturients to the anaesthetic staff allows the development of a management plan and means that all staffs are aware of a high-risk patient.

PATHOPHYSIOLOGY

MH represents a metabolic event, rather than a specific genetic entity, where there is a common pathway of excessive release of intracellular calcium from the sarcoplasmic reticulum of muscle cells. As a result, there is uncontrolled, increased muscle metabolism with muscle rigidity, a progressive rise in temperature, and biochemical indicators of hypermetabolism with acidosis, hypercarbia and hyperkalaemia (see Table 13.1). In severe reactions, there is extensive muscle damage with myoglobinuria, which can cause acute renal failure and disseminated intravascular coagulation.

MANAGEMENT OPTIONS AND DISCUSSION

Laboratory diagnosis of malignant hyperpyrexia

Despite efforts to find a non-invasive diagnostic test, the *in vitro* muscle contraction tests (IVCTs) of skeletal muscle strips have been used to diagnose MHS for over 20 years. Testing is carried out at specialist centres of which there is only one

Table 13.1 – Clinical features of MH.

1. Rise in core temperature of 1–2°C/h
2. Hypercarbia
3. Tachycardia and cardiac arrhythmias
4. Metabolic acidosis
5. Hypoxaemia
6. Hyperkalaemia
7. Failure of jaw relaxation following suxamethonium
8. Muscle rigidity of some muscle groups
9. Rise in serum creatinine kinase
10. Myoglobinuria and renal failure
11. Disseminated intravascular coagulation

in the UK – the Leeds MH Investigation Unit. The patient is referred to the unit where a muscle biopsy is performed using a femoral nerve block with an amide local anaesthetic agent. Muscle is excised from the vastus muscle. Tests involve separate *in vitro* exposure of the muscle to halothane and caffeine, and the measurement of the tension generated in response to both drugs. Muscle strips from MHS individuals will produce an increase in tension at a lower concentration of both halothane and caffeine than normal muscle. In cases where the muscle reacts normally to one of the drugs but not the other a MM equivocal (MHE) diagnosis is assigned. This group of patients is then treated in the same manner as the MHS group. Muscle that contracts normally is assigned a MM negative diagnosis (MHN). These results conform to a protocol standardised by the European Malignant Hyperpyrexia Group in 1983 (see The European Malignant Hyperpyrexia Group in Further reading). The MHE group of patients will include individuals who do not have a genetic predisposition to the disorder.

The lack of specificity of both tests, and the lack of sensitivity of the caffeine test, has stimulated research to improve the accuracy of phenotyping necessary for genetic studies of MH. Two drugs, ryanodine and chlorocresol, that induce *in vitro* muscle contracture have been investigated. The predictive probability of various contracture tests in determining MHS has been examined. The rank order of correlation with MH diagnosis of the tests studied was: ryanodine > dynamic halothane > static halothane > caffeine test. This suggests that an additional ryanodine contracture test may be useful in discriminating between MHS and normal individuals. A preservative in some pharmaceutical preparations, 4-chloro-m-cresol (4-CmC), affects the calcium ion release channel of skeletal muscle sarcoplasmic reticulum and causes muscle contracture. It may also prove useful in phenotyping in the future.

Molecular genetics of malignant hyperpyrexia

Genetic linkage of the gene conferring susceptibility to MH with the region of chromosome 19q close to the gene encoding the ryanodine receptor (RYR1) was first published in two reports in 1990. The abnormalities in MHS muscle lie in the regulation of myoplasmic calcium. Calcium is stored mainly in the sarcoplasmic reticulum of skeletal muscle and is released by excitation–contraction coupling. The RYR (ryanodine receptor) is a protein containing a calcium-release channel in the sarcoplasmic reticulum of skeletal muscle.

Early studies found linkage to chromosome 19q12.1–13.2, the locus of the RYR gene, which encodes the skeletal muscle sarcoplasmic reticulum calcium-release channel. The genetics of human MH, however, has proved more complex. Less than 60 families worldwide have been large enough to provide useful genetic data. Results have demonstrated genetic heterogeneity with study results showing 30–80% of families consistent with linkage to the RYR1. Development in the search for mutations of RYR1 has occurred and at least 20 mutations have been found in these families, but there is a high incidence of these mutations not being co-inherited with the disorder. Where linkage data has excluded the RYR1 locus, several other genetic loci have been investigated including mutant alleles at loci on chromosomes 1q (dihydropyridine-sensitive L-type calcium channel-A1S), 3q 5p 7q (dihydropyridine-sensitive L-type calcium channel-LA2).

Central core disease (CCD) is a dominantly inherited myopathy in which affected individuals may show delayed motor milestones in infancy or muscle weakness in the lower limbs. Patients are often not diagnosed until later in life because of the slow or non-progressive clinical course of CCD. It, too, is due to a mutation in the RYR1. Histochemical and electron microscopic examination of muscle shows well demarcated, centrally-located cores, with a predominance of type 1 fibres. Some individuals in central-core families may be diagnosed as MHS but have normal muscle histology. Not all individuals with CCD are susceptible to MH. All members of central-core families should be regarded as susceptible to MH and have their MH status investigated.

It is well known that MHS individuals can be anaesthetised with triggering agents and not develop MH. Additional factors may influence the probability of developing a fulminant MH syndrome in individuals who are heterozygous with respect to MH predisposition. These could include the physiological state of the muscles when exposed to triggering agents and the degree of activation of the sympathetic nervous system.

Clinical features and management

The features of an MH reaction are hypermetabolism, muscle rigidity and muscle breakdown. It is important that anaesthetists are aware of this condition, as volatile agents and suxamethonium are known triggers. It is necessary to plan a safe approach to normal and operative delivery for patients with the condition.

It has now been established that amide local anaesthetic agents are safe and therefore regional anaesthesia is preferred; epidurals and spinals can be used as the need indicates. Epidurals in labour reduce the release of catecholamines, cortisol and other hormones. Although there is little evidence to suggest stress can trigger an MH reaction, it would seem appropriate to obtund any stress response. There was some doubt as to the safety of vasopressors as it was thought that the sympathomimetic effects could trigger a reaction. Ephedrine has now been used safely. Monitoring should involve frequent measurement of temperature and should continue into the post-delivery period as a case has been reported of MH presenting in the recovery period.

General anaesthesia should be avoided unless regional anaesthesia fails or is contraindicated. However, there should be a contingency plan for general anaesthesia if required in an emergency. Hence, there should be a careful assessment of the airway and routine antacid prophylaxis should be given. An anaesthetic machine which has been flushed for 20 min with 100% oxygen at 10 l/min and has had all the tubing changed with a fresh CO_2 absorbent, is deemed to be safe for use. The general anaesthetic should involve the use of non-triggering drugs (see Table 13.2). A modified rapid sequence induction is required to avoid the use of suxamethonium. The patient is pre-oxygenated and monitoring established to include direct arterial pressure and core temperature. The patient is induced with alfentanil 1–2 mg, propofol 2.5 mg/kg, and rocuronium 0.9 mg/kg with cricoid pressure applied. When relaxation has occurred, the patient's trachea is intubated. Cricoid pressure is removed when the anaesthetist is sure the tracheal tube is in the correct position. Anaesthesia is maintained with a propofol target infusion. A 50% mixture of nitrous oxide in oxygen is used until delivery. Oxytocin is regarded as safe and can be given as usual to help contract the uterus following delivery. Morphine may be used for pain relief and the muscle relaxation reversed with a routine dose of neostigmine and glycopyrronium.

The current trend is not to pre-treat with dantrolene. Apart from the unpleasant side effects of weakness and nausea, it has been associated with uterine atony leading to excessive bleeding.

Table 13.2 – Trigger drugs for MH.

Drugs known to trigger MH	Drugs thought to be safe
All volatile anaesthetic agents Suxamethonium	Nitrous oxide Non-depolarizing neuromuscular blocking drugs Neostigmine Atropine and glycopyrronium Barbiturates, propofol, benzodiazepines Amide local anaesthetics Opioids Droperidol Metoclopramide

Management of a malignant hyperpyrexia reaction

Anaesthetists must always be aware of the possibility of an undiagnosed case. Occasionally, a 'routine' pre-operative biochemical screen will reveal an increased serum creatinine kinase concentration in an apparently asymptomatic patient. The difficulty is that there is no specific sign and the diagnosis is often the recognition of several signs occurring in a pattern. A first indication is jaw rigidity following suxamethonium. After this, the signs of hypermetabolism can be seen – increasing temperature, heart rate and end-tidal carbon dioxide.

The differential diagnoses are:

1. Inadequate analgesia/anaesthesia

2. Inappropriate circuit/ventilation/fresh gas flow

3. Sepsis

4. Endocrine conditions – thyroid storm, phaeochromocytoma

5. Anaphylaxis

6. Cerebral ischaemia

If MH is suspected, it must be treated promptly as the mortality rate without treatment is very high.

The treatment of an MH reaction consists of:

1. Discontinuing volatile agent and using high flow oxygen to ventilate the patient

2. Maintaining anaesthesia using a propofol infusion

3. Commencing active cooling – remove excessive drapes, cold intravenous solutions (do not give any containing calcium), ice can be packed into the groins and axillae and body cavities can be irrigated with cold solutions

4. The definitive treatment is dantrolene 2.5 mg/kg up to a maximum of 10 mg/kg. Dantrolene should be available where general anaesthetics are given. Dantrolene limits the build up of calcium ions within muscle cells, thus decreasing intracellular calcium and so decreasing the effects seen with MH. It should be given until the rise in temperature, heart rate and carbon dioxide subsides. Doses may need to be repeated at a later time if a recrudescence of the reaction occurs, particularly as blood levels of dantrolene decrease.

5. Acidosis and hyperkalaemia should be treated.

6. Urine output should be maintained as the release of myoglobin can damage renal tubules if allowed to accumulate. It should be noted that an ampoule of dantrolene contains 3 g mannitol.

7. Coagulopathies may be seen and should be corrected.

8. Post-operative care should be in an intensive care unit.

Foetal malignant hyperpyrexia

There is a further consideration with regard to obstetric anaesthesia and MH. The mother herself may not have the disorder but her partner may and as the inheritance is autosomal dominant, the baby may be susceptible. Volatile agents cross the placenta and placental transfer of suxamethonium occurs, and a case of a baby being born with a presumptive MH reaction has been reported. In such a case, the mother should have a trigger free anaesthetic and the paediatricians should be alerted to the possible problem.

KEY LEARNING POINTS

1. In a busy obstetric unit there will be women or their partners who have been diagnosed as MHS. It is important that these cases are identified and referred early in the pregnancy for anaesthetic assessment.

2. Once a suitable care plan has been made, it should be documented in the patient's notes and be readily accessible in the delivery suite.

3. Regional anaesthesia is safe and is preferred but there should be a contingency plan for carrying out safe general anaesthesia should it be necessary.

4. Anaesthetists must be alert to the presenting features of MH and know how to treat it.

Further reading

Beebe JJ, Sessler DI. Preparation of anaesthetic machines for patients susceptible to malignant hyperpyrexia. *Anesthesiology* 1988; **66**: 395–400.

Cass N, Cass L. *Pharmacology for Anaesthetists.* Churchill Livingstone, Edinburgh, 1994.

Denborough MA. Malignant hyperthermia. *Lancet* 1998; **352**: 1131–6.

Fagerlund TH, Islander G, Twetman ER, Berg K. Malignant hyperthermia susceptibility, an autosomal dominant disorder? *Clinical Genetics* 1997; **51**: 365–9.

Hopkins PM. Malignant hyperthermia. *Royal College of Anaesthetists Newsletter* 1999; **46**: 99–103.

Hopkins PM. Malignant hyperthermia: advances in clinical management and diagnosis. *British Journal of Anaesthesia* 2000; **85**: 118–28.

Lucy SJ. Anaesthesia for Caesarean delivery of a malignant hyperpyrexia susceptible parturient. *Canadian Journal of Anaesthesia* 1994; **41**: 1220–6.

MHAUS. Professional Advisory council adopts new policy statement on local anaesthetics. *MHAUS Communicator Spring* 1985; III(4).

Pollock N, Langton E. Management of malignant hyperthermia susceptible parturients. *Anaesthesia and Intensive Care* 1997; **25**: 398–407.

The European Malignant Hyperpyrexia Group. A protocol for the investigation of malignant hyperpyrexia (MH) susceptibility. *British Journal of Anaesthesia* 1984; **56**: 1267–9.

Updated technical bulletin for malignant hyperpyrexia. *American Society of Anesthesiologists Newsletter* 1992; **56**: 30–1.

14

OBSTETRIC PATIENTS WITH ORGAN TRANSPLANTS

C. Mendonca and P. Clyburn

CASE HISTORY

A 35-year-old, gravida 3, para 0, insulin-dependent diabetic presented at 30 weeks of gestation to the obstetric anaesthesia clinic. The patient had received a renal transplant 5 years previously for end-stage renal failure secondary to diabetes mellitus. She was initially immunosuppressed with tacrolimus, azathioprine and prednisolone, but prednisolone was discontinued 1 year post transplant. She had been hypertensive for 10 years, but her blood pressure was well controlled with clonidine. She was on a twice-daily combination of actrapid and monotard insulin to control her diabetes. She did not have any history of rejection or infectious complications. Her renal transplant surgery was complicated by fluid overload, which required admission to the intensive care for postoperative ventilation. As a result, she was terrified of general anaesthesia and was noted to have poor venous access.

She first became pregnant 18 months after her renal transplantation, but the pregnancy resulted in a stillbirth at 25 weeks gestation. Her second pregnancy, 6 months later, ended with a miscarriage at 18 weeks.

She was generally well during this, her third pregnancy, and although she usually became short of breath on moderate exercise, this had not deteriorated during the pregnancy. Her insulin requirements had increased during the second trimester and she also needed increases in the dose of tacrolimus (3 mg/day until 20 weeks to 5 mg/day at 32 weeks). At 31 weeks, she was commenced on atenolol to help to control her hypertension. She developed mild proteinuria at 33 weeks, although she maintained good urine output throughout her pregnancy. Laboratory tests at 34 weeks showed a haemoglobin of 10.8 g/dl, platelets 231×10^9/l, white cell count 14.2×10^9/l, a slightly raised blood urea (8.1 mmol/l) and serum creatinine (135 μmol/l).

In view of her poor obstetric history, the obstetricians decided on an elective Caesarean section at 38 weeks gestation. The anaesthetic plan was to perform this under regional anaesthesia. At 34 weeks gestation, a foetal cardiotocogram was abnormal with late decelerations suggesting foetal distress. She, therefore, underwent urgent Caesarean section under spinal anaesthesia. The intra-operative course was uneventful and she gave birth to a live infant. During the peri-operative period, her blood glucose was maintained at normal levels with intravenous glucose and insulin infusions. Her renal function remained stable during the peri-operative period. She was discharged home on day 6 after the Caesarean section. She was regularly reviewed in the nephrology clinic, and a year following delivery her renal function remained stable.

DESCRIPTION OF THE PROBLEM

This case illustrates the various issues that need to be addressed in the management of a pregnant mother with a renal transplant.

- With increasing numbers of renal transplants being carried out in women of child-bearing age, pregnancy in a renal transplant patient is no longer a rare event.

- Chronic renal failure is associated with infertility and menstrual irregularity due to hypogonadotrophic hypogonadism. Renal transplant is the only hope for a successful pregnancy in many women with chronic renal disease.

- The major problems that are encountered are:
  - the physiological changes of pregnancy on renal function and
  - the potential problems of immunosuppressant drugs.

PATHOPHYSIOLOGY

During pregnancy, renal blood flow increases by about 80% over the non-pregnant levels, which is achieved by the middle of the second trimester. The glomerular filtration rate and creatinine clearance increase by 50%. These important changes in glomerular filtration may adversely affect the long-term graft survival. Crowe *et al.* studied the obstetric data and renal parameters in 33 pregnancies following renal transplantation and found that the majority of them delivered prematurely with a mean gestational age of 34.2 weeks. The mean serum creatinine and creatinine clearance remained stable throughout the pregnancy, but there was a significant increase in proteinuria at delivery, which resolved within 3 months after delivery.

Premature labour and delivery is a common obstetric complication; the incidence varies between 20–59%, with impaired renal function and elevated blood pressure resulting in low birth weight. Corticosteroid therapy is also associated with premature rupture of membranes, which can lead to premature delivery. The factors adversely affecting the outcome of pregnancy are shorter time interval between transplant and conception, pre-pregnancy hypertension, diabetes, chronic renal insufficiency and high immunosuppressive drug dosage.

MANAGEMENT OPTIONS AND DISCUSSION

Immunosuppression therapy

Cyclosporin, tacrolimus, azathioprine and corticosteroids are frequently used for immunosuppression following renal transplantation. Cyclosporin crosses the placenta from mother to foetus in a ratio of 1 : 1 and has been reported to be associated with intra-uterine growth retardation. Cyclosporin and tacrolimus requirements increase during pregnancy, mainly because of increased blood volume and altered metabolism. Hence, serum concentration of these drugs should be frequently monitored to ensure correct therapeutic levels. Hypertension is commonly observed in pregnant patients taking cyclosporin; it decreases endogenous nitric oxide production and increases systemic vascular resistance. Furthermore, the incidence of pre-eclampsia is higher in patients taking cyclosporin compared to the general obstetric population, and an incidence of 33% has been reported. Intra-uterine growth retardation has been associated with cyclosporin use. Tacrolimus has a similar mode of action to cyclosporin, but the incidence of hypertension and pre-eclampsia is lower than with cyclosporin and is increasingly used in these patients.

Azathioprine produces dose-dependent myelotoxicity. It may cause megaloblastic anaemia and thrombocytopaenia. Neonatal leukopaenia and thrombocytopaenia has been reported in infants born to mothers treated with azathioprine. As these immunosuppressant drugs are excreted in breast milk, breast-feeding is best avoided following delivery.

Exogenous steroid therapy has been associated with premature rupture of membranes and intra-uterine growth retardation. When used in high doses, steroids can worsen glucose intolerance associated with the pregnancy itself as well as making the management of the diabetic mother more difficult. The long-term use of steroids can also result in fluid retention and weight gain.

The incidence of graft rejection during pregnancy is similar to non-pregnant transplant patients. Graft survival and long-term renal function are not affected by pregnancy, provided that pregnancy is initiated in patients with normal and stable renal function.

Management of delivery

Normal vaginal delivery is possible following renal transplantation as the renal allograft is typically implanted in the iliac fossa and does not interfere with a vaginal delivery. However, the associated intra-uterine growth retardation, high blood pressure and deterioration in renal function may lead to early Caesarean section. Pelvic osteodystrophy secondary to prior chronic renal failure and steroid therapy may also result in disproportion between the foetus and the pelvis.

Anaesthetic management is similar to the normal pregnant patient provided renal function and blood pressure are normal. Initial laboratory tests should include full blood count, serum electrolytes, urea, creatinine and glucose. Plasma levels of immunosuppressant drugs should be regularly monitored. Regular ultrasound scans allow the evaluation of foetal growth. As these patients are at risk of sepsis, strict aseptic technique should be maintained during intravascular cannulation and the performance of regional techniques.

As these patients are susceptible to hypertension and pre-eclampsia, assessment of platelet count and clotting studies should be performed prior to surgery. If parameters are within normal limits, it is acceptable to use any appropriate regional technique.

If general anaesthesia is employed, it is important to appropriately obtund the intubation and extubation response. It is also very important to monitor the urine output closely, as renal function may suddenly worsen if the mother becomes dehydrated.

LIVER TRANSPLANT

Although renal transplantation is by far the most common transplant the obstetric anaesthetist will encounter, there are increasing numbers of women with other transplants who may become pregnant.

Liver size and morphology do not change during pregnancy. Although cardiac output is significantly increased during pregnancy, there is actually a net decrease in the proportion of cardiac output going to the liver because of diversion to the uteroplacental unit. Enzyme levels will be altered and alkaline phosphatase levels can increase by 2–4-fold, while there may be a slight increase in lactate dehydrogenase and bilirubin. These normal physiological changes make it difficult to detect episodes of transplant rejection in pregnancy. Mild to moderate renal insufficiency has been reported in pregnant mothers with liver transplants. Cyclosporin and tacrolimus cause systemic and afferent renal arteriolar vasoconstriction by increasing the production of thromboxane A_2 and by interfering with nitric oxide-mediated vasodilatation. These changes can result in a significant reduction in glomerular filtration rate and renal blood flow. Pregnancy may be complicated by pre-eclampsia, anaemia, intra-uterine growth retardation and pre-term delivery. These changes are mainly related to hypertension and renal insufficiency, caused by the immunosuppressant drugs.

The hyperdynamic state of chronic liver disease persists in some patients, even after the orthotopic liver transplantation. An abnormally elevated cardiac output has been observed during the first trimester and early second trimester. A hyperdynamic circulation with increased cardiac output and compensatory vasodilatation causes endothelial activation and injury that can contribute to the development of pre-eclampsia. Stable renal function and adequate control of blood pressure in these mothers improves the outcome of pregnancy.

The recommended interval from transplantation to conception is at least 9–12 months, which allows stabilisation of hepatic function and treatment of opportunistic infections. Pregnancy does not increase the likelihood of graft rejection. There is an increased incidence of premature delivery by Caesarean section, related to obstetric problems, such as pregnancy-induced hypertension.

CARDIAC TRANSPLANT

The transplanted heart is devoid of any innervation and, therefore, is not under endogenous autonomic nervous system control. Drugs acting on the vagus nerve (e.g. atropine) do not produce any chronotropic effect. Only direct acting sympathomemitic drugs (e.g. isoprenaline) reliably produce chronotropic or inotropic effects. Over time, there is up-regulation of beta-receptors, which become more sensitive to catecholamines. Despite this, the normal physiological increases in haemodynamic parameters of pregnancy still occur. The enlarged blood volume of pregnancy, usually in the order of 40%, increases the stroke volume by means of the Starling mechanism, which remains intact in the transplanted heart.

Maternal and foetal complications are similar to those of patients with renal and liver transplant, such as a high incidence of hypertension, although normal vaginal delivery has been reported following heart transplantation. Pregnancy itself does not increase the incidence of acute rejection.

During pre-anaesthetic assessment, special attention should be given to exercise tolerance during pregnancy after transplantation. Recent cardiac catheterisation reports and echocardiography are useful in evaluating left ventricular function. Coronary atherosclerosis may be accelerated in transplanted hearts and problems, such as myocardial ischaemia, may be asymptomatic due to the complete denervation of the heart.

Epidural analgesia using a low concentration of local anaesthetic and an opioid is a good choice for pain relief during labour. Combined spinal and epidural anaesthesia with small doses of local anaesthetic in the subarachnoid space followed by gradual extension of the regional blockade with epidural top ups will have the benefit of maintaining cardiovascular stability for Caesarean section.

KEY LEARNING POINTS

1. Pregnancy should be deferred for at least 12 months after any organ transplant to allow stable graft function and immunosuppressive regimen to be established.

2. Pregnancy in transplant recipients should be considered high risk and requires a multidisciplinary approach.

3. During the pregnancy, the mother should be carefully screened for the development of pre-eclampsia, gestational diabetes, infections and renal insufficiency.

4. Immunosuppression therapy should be constantly monitored to avoid graft rejection and drug toxicity.

5. There is considerable neonatal morbidity in terms of prematurity, IUGR and low birth weight.

6. Pregnancy-induced hypertension is more common in all transplant recipients.

7. Pregnancy does not appear to have any deleterious effect on graft survival.

8. Since immunosuppressive drugs may be excreted in the breast milk, it is safer to advise against breast-feeding.

Further reading

Carr DB, Larson AM, Schmucker BC, *et al.* Maternal haemodynamics and pregnancy outcome in women with prior orthotopic liver transplantation. *Liver Transplantation* 2000; **6**: 213–21.

Casele HL, Laifer SA. Association of pregnancy complications and choice of immunosuppressant in liver transplant patients. *Transplantation* 1998; **65**: 581–2.

Crowe AV, Rustom R, Gradden C, *et al.* Pregnancy does not adversely affect the renal transplant function. *Quarterly Journal of Medicine* 1999; **92**: 631–5.

Muirhead N, Sabharwal AR, Rieder MJ, *et al.* The outcome of pregnancy following renal transplantation. The experience of single centre. *Transplantation* 1992; **54**: 429–32.

Poole JH. Liver transplant and pregnancy. *Journal of Perinatal and Neonatal Nursing* 1997; **11**: 25–34.

Rieu P, Neyrat N, Hiesse C, Charpentier B. Thirty three pregnancies in a population of 1725 renal transplant patients. *Transplantation Proceedings* 1997; **29**: 2459–60.

Shen AY-J, Mansukhani PW. Is pregnancy contraindicated after cardiac transplantation? A case report and literature review. *International Journal of Cardiology* 1997; **60**: 151–6.

Tanabe K, Kobayashi C, Takahashi K, *et al.* Long term renal function after pregnancy in renal transplant recipients. *Transplantation Proceedings* 1997; **29**: 1567–8.

Touraine JL, Audra Ph, Lefrancois N, *et al.* Pregnancy in renal transplant patients: 45 case reports. *Transplantation Proceedings* 1997; **29**: 2472–4.

15

POST-DURAL PUNCTURE HEADACHE

C. Busby and P. Clyburn

CASE HISTORY

A 29-year-old parturient, gravida 2, para 1, requested epidural analgesia following spontaneous onset of labour at 41 weeks gestation. The pregnancy had been uncomplicated, she was fit and well and a trial of labour was planned. Three years previously, she had uneventful epidural analgesia for labour, which was successfully extended for lower segment Caesarean section following a delayed first stage of labour.

On this occasion, she was admitted to the delivery suite in labour and within an hour she requested epidural analgesia. The obstetric anaesthetist, a junior trainee, was unable to locate the epidural space despite several attempts. A senior trainee successfully placed an epidural catheter, which threaded easily. Aspiration for blood and cerebrospinal fluid (CSF) was negative; however, an exaggerated response to the initial test dose (10 ml bupivacaine 0.1% + fentanyl 2 μg/ml) was noted. Six hours later, the patient required a Caesarean section for delayed first stage of labour. A dense block to the level of the T2 dermatome was achieved (using loss of sensation to ice) after only 7.5 ml bupivacaine 0.5%. Following this, the possibility of accidental dural puncture (ADP) was discussed with the patient.

On the first day post-partum, the patient started to complain of headache. This failed to respond to simple analgesia and rehydration. By the second day, it had increased in severity and was postural in nature. Post-dural puncture headache (PDPH) and the treatment options were again discussed with the patient, who declined an epidural blood patch (EBP) at this stage. A single dose of adrenocorticotrophic hormone (ACTH) 1 mg was administered by intramuscular injection, but there was no improvement. By that evening, the patient became quite distressed and requested an EBP. Unfortunately, she was now pyrexial. Blood cultures were taken, she was commenced on broad-spectrum antibiotics (co-amoxiclav and gentamicin) and within 24 h she was afebrile. A consultant anaesthetist performed an EBP on the third post-partum day. Autologous blood 15 ml was injected into the epidural space and 10 ml was sent for culture. The patient was allowed to mobilise after 4 h. There was immediate, long-lasting relief of her headache from this procedure and she was able to go home later the same day.

DEFINITION OF THE PROBLEM

PDPH was recognised by August Bier, who performed the first spinal anaesthetic over 100 years ago. Headache is a relatively common complication of both intentional dural puncture (spinal anaesthesia, diagnostic or therapeutic lumbar puncture, myelography, etc.) and ADP (during attempted epidural cannulation).

- The incidence of PDPH is about 1% in obstetric patients following spinal anaesthesia using fine bore (24 G or smaller) pencil-point needles, compared with up to 30% in patients following lumbar puncture with 20 G sharp bevelled (Quinke) needles.

- ADP occurs during 0.5–2.5% of epidural insertions and is followed by a headache in around 70% of cases.

PATHOPHYSIOLOGY

A hole in the dura allows persistent leakage of CSF, reducing the volume and pressure in the subarachnoid space. This leads to traction on the meninges and blood vessels, which are richly innervated by pain fibres, an effect that is increased by gravity when the subject assumes an upright position. Compensatory vasodilatation occurs in response to the loss of CSF and is thought to contribute to the sensation of pain by a similar mechanism to migraine. This is the rationale for the use of the anti-migraine drug sumatriptan, a $5-HT_1$ agonist, which has been used with some success in the treatment of PDPH.

MANAGEMENT OPTIONS AND DISCUSSION

Following ADP with a 16 G Tuohy needle, a significant headache occurs in 60–90% of patients. ADP may be detected immediately by the free flow of CSF through the Tuohy needle when the stylet is withdrawn. CSF can be distinguished from saline by the presence of glucose, easily detected by a 'BM stick'. In this case, ADP was not obvious at the time of epidural insertion, but was suspected by a greater than normal response to the test dose of local anaesthetic, suggesting a partial subarachnoid block. This may have been due to trauma to the dura by the hypodermic needle used for subcutaneous tissue infiltration at the start of the procedure (more likely in a slim patient in whom the epidural space may be relatively superficial), or due to a partial tear of the dura by either the Tuohy needle or the epidural catheter.

The case illustrates the need for cautious administration and monitoring of the response to initial and subsequent doses of local anaesthetic in any patient receiving epidural anaesthesia. Obstetric patients about to undergo spinal or epidural anaesthesia should be warned of the possibility of PDPH as part of obtaining informed consent, since any significant complication with a rate of 1% or more is common enough so that it should be mentioned to all patients.

Differential diagnosis

Headache is a common symptom in the early postpartum period and is usually unrelated to anaesthetic intervention. Differential diagnosis includes common, relatively trivial causes, such as exhaustion, anxiety, dehydration, simple tension headache and migraine, as well as more serious pathology including meningitis, pre-eclampsia and intracranial haemorrhage, infarction or a space-occupying lesion.

In many patients who develop a characteristic PDPH, there is no record of an obvious dural puncture. It must be assumed that either the puncture went undetected or that the Tuohy needle damaged the dura but the subarachnoid membrane remained intact initially but subsequently broke down and leaked CSF. Therefore, the absence of a recognised dural puncture does not exclude the possibility of PDPH.

Features

PDPH is typically postural (relieved by lying flat and exacerbated by the upright posture). It is usually frontal or fronto-occipital and is often described as dull or throbbing in nature. Pain can radiate to the neck, back or shoulders. Associated symptoms include nausea and vomiting, neck stiffness, visual disturbances, tinnitus, deafness and other cranial nerve dysfunction. The headache is of variable severity, and in up to a third of patients, is incapacitating. Onset is also variable, usually 24–48-h post-puncture; however, the headache can start immediately or be delayed for several days (when the patient might have already been discharged from hospital). PDPH is usually a self-limiting condition lasting 2–10 days, though rarely, if left untreated, can persist as chronic headache for as long as a year or more. Other important sequelae include seizures and subarachnoid, subdural or extradural haemorrhage. Even death from bilateral subdural haematoma following lumbar puncture has been described. Fortunately, such occurrences are rare.

Risk factors

PDPH is reportedly higher in young slim women, especially if there is a predisposition to headaches, and following early mobilisation, though not in pregnancy *per se*. The size and shape of the hole in the dura is also important. Previously, it was believed that pencil-point needles (e.g. Whitacre and Sprotte needles) parted the dural fibres atraumatically, while sharp-bevelled needles (e.g. Quincke needles) cut the fibres leaving a more distinct hole and allowing greater loss of CSF. This has been challenged by recent electron micrographs of cadaveric pig dura after puncture by both types of needle, which reveal that pencil-point needles actually appear to cause a more disorganised, ragged hole. It is proposed that this may stimulate an inflammatory reaction that seals the defect more rapidly than the clean, surgical incision made by Quinke needles.

Prevention of post-dural puncture headache

The rate of PDPH following deliberate dural puncture for spinal anaesthesia is decreased by the use of smaller gauge needles, with pencil-point or bullet-shaped tips, as discussed previously.

The incidence of ADP during epidural insertion is dependant on operator experience and technique. It is reduced by adequate training and supervision of anaesthetic trainees, particularly during their first 10–20 epidural insertions when the risk is highest. The use of loss of resistance to saline rather than air allows continuous pressure on the syringe plunger and is associated with a lower rate of ADP as well as having other advantages. Similarly, it has been suggested that the use of the paramedian rather than the midline approach to the epidural space may reduce the chance of dural puncture (DP). Orientating the bevel of the Tuohy needle (so it is parallel with the longitudinal fibres of the dura) is associated with a lower rate of headache if the dura is punctured, possibly because this causes a smaller dural tear. The technique of needle insertion with the bevel facing laterally, however, necessitates rotation of the needle by 90° to allow catheter placement. This action may tear the dural fibres causing an increased rate of ADP and, therefore, needle rotation is not advisable.

MANAGEMENT OF ACCIDENTAL DURAL PUNCTURE

If dural puncture is recognised, the catheter can be threaded intrathecally and used as such. This prevents the need for another attempt at epidural placement, which risks a further dural puncture; also the presence of the catheter may promote a localised inflammatory response with earlier plugging of the defect once it is removed. Patient and staff need to be warned about the use of an intrathecal catheter and it must be clearly labelled (Table 15.1). Intrathecal analgesia is then established with intermittent boluses of low dose local anaesthetic and opioid

Table 15.1 – Management following ADP.

Early
? Avoid excessive pushing in second stage
Give full explanation to patient
Allow normal mobilisation
Encourage hydration
Prescribe simple analgesics and laxatives post-delivery
? Epidural infusion of 1 l normal saline in 24 h following delivery
If develops PDPH
Explain and discuss EBP. If patient reluctant to have EBP (especially if headache not incapacitating):
Simple analgesia and caffeine
Try intramuscular ACTH 1 mg
Try subcutaneous sumatriptan 6 mg

(e.g. 2–3 mg bupivacaine plus 10–20 µg fentanyl). Alternatively, epidural analgesia may be performed at an adjacent spinal interspace. Once the mother is comfortable, a full explanation should be offered.

Measures to decrease the risk of developing headache, or at least its severity, following recognised dural puncture include:

- Encouraging adequate (though not over) hydration.

- Prevention of prolonged expulsive efforts during the second stage of labour. This is controversial as it merely delays the onset of headache without decreasing its incidence, while increasing the rate of instrumental delivery. A recent retrospective study of patients who had an ADP, found that women who had Caesarean section before full cervical dilatation were less likely to develop PDPH than women who pushed in the second stage.

- Infusion of 1 l of normal saline through the epidural catheter over 24 h. There is some evidence that this too only delays the onset of headache without influencing its incidence.

- Prophylactic EBP via the epidural catheter. This is controversial as it is claimed that early blood patch is less effective than when performed after 24 h and is also unnecessary in those patients who would not have developed headache.

- Laxatives to prevent straining due to constipation.

Use of abdominal binders is no longer recommended, although transient relief of the headache by abdominal compression can be used as a diagnostic indicator. Enforced bed rest is also discouraged, because of increased risk of thromboembolism.

MANAGEMENT OF ESTABLISHED PDPH

Diagnosis of PDPH is usually straightforward, based on the characteristic features in association with known or suspected ADP. The cause of the headache and various treatment options should be discussed with the patient. Depending on initial headache severity, management can be initially conservative, and in addition to the above measures, includes the use of simple analgesics (such as paracetamol and non-steroidal anti-inflammatory drugs and weak opioids, such as codeine phosphate).

Other drugs that have been tried with variable success include sumatriptan (6 mg by subcutaneous injection), ACTH (1 mg by intramuscular injection or an intravenous infusion of 1.5 IU/kg) and caffeine tablets (300 mg orally in the morning).

If the headache is severe, or fails to respond, EBP should be offered.

Epidural blood patch

Although invasive, EBP is considered by many to be the treatment of choice for PDPH. It consists of injection of 10–20 ml of autologous blood into the epidural space. Relief is usually immediate; magnetic resonance imaging following EBP confirms that initially, this is due to cranial displacement of CSF by the mass of epidural blood, which over the next few hours disperses, leaving a thin layer of haematoma adherent to the dura. This presumably seals the defect accounting for the long-term success of the technique.

Initial success of EBP is of the order of 90%, though some of these patients relapse after 1–2 days, requiring a repeat blood patch. More than two blood patches are not recommended. Overall, long-term relief following single blood patch is probably achieved in 60–75% of patients.

Contraindications to EBP are the same as for other neuroaxial procedures and include patient refusal, coagulopathy and local or systemic sepsis. In the febrile patient, such as in this case, EBP is usually delayed until the temperature has settled.

Conduct of EBP requires an experienced anaesthetist to identify the epidural space. Ideally, the space below that at which the dural puncture occurred is chosen, because the injected blood has been observed to spread mainly in a cranial direction. Once the epidural space has been located, an assistant withdraws 15–20 ml of venous blood from the patient, in an aseptic manner. The blood (10–20 ml) is then injected slowly into the epidural space, or less if the patient complains of back or leg pain. The remainder of the blood is traditionally retained for culture. Discomfort is common during the injection and up to a quarter of patients complain of short-term backache afterwards. There is also a small, but real, risk of repeat dural puncture, especially if the anatomy is abnormal in some way. Fortunately, there appears to be no effect on future epidural analgesia.

KEY LEARNING POINTS

1. PDPH is a relatively common and distressing condition.

2. The headache is characteristic and typically postural.

3. When it occurs, PDPH should be diagnosed and treated appropriately. Patients must be kept under close review until cured and encouraged to report any reccurrence.

4. Its incidence can be minimised by the use of fine gauge (25 G or finer), pencil-point needles for spinal anaesthesia and by good training of epidural technique.

5. PDPH is usually self-limiting, but can occasionally lead to serious complications if not treated appropriately.

6. EBP is an effective treatment for the majority.

Further reading

Angle P, Thompson D, Halpern S, Wilson DB. Second stage pushing correlates with headache after unintentional dural puncture in parturients. *Canadian Journal of Anaesthesia* 1999; **46**: 861–86.

Cowan CM, Moore EW. A survey of epidural technique and accidental dural puncture rates among obstetric anaesthetists. *International Journal of Obstetric Anesthesia* 2001; **10**: 11–16.

Duffy PJ, Crosby ET. The epidural blood patch. Resolving the controversies. *Canadian Journal of Anaesthesia* 1999; **46**: 878–86.

Jeskins GD, Moore PAS, Cooper GM, Lewis M. Long term morbidity following dural puncture in an obstetric population. *International Journal of Obstetric Anesthesia* 2001; **10**: 17–24.

Reina MA, Leon-Casasola OA, Lopez A, Andres J, Martin S, Mora M. An *in vitro* study of dural lesions produced by 25 gauge Quincke and Whitacre needles evaluated by scanning electron microscopy. *Regional Anesthesia and Pain Medicine* 2000; **25**: 393–402.

Reynolds F. Dural puncture and headache. *British Medical Journal* 1993; **306**: 874–6.

Vakharia SB, Thomas PS, Rosenbaum AE, Wasenko JJ, Fellows DG. Magnetic resonance imaging of cerebrospinal fluid leak and tamponade effect of blood patch in post dural puncture headache. *Anesthesia and Analgesia* 1997; **84**: 585–90.

16

PRE–ECLAMPSIA AND ECLAMPSIA

M.J. Evans

CASE HISTORY

A 17-year-old, previously well primigravida was admitted at 28 weeks gestation with lethargy and reduced foetal movements. On examination, she looked unwell but was apyrexial, weighed 100 kg and her height was 163 cm. Her blood pressure was 130/85 mmHg, and she had oedema of her ankles and fingers. Her respiratory rate was 20/min and breath sounds were vesicular. She was alert and had no neurological signs. Biochemical profile showed, normal electrolytes, urea 4.5 mmol/l, creatinine 85 μmol/l, albumin 30 g/l, uric acid 0.38 mmol/l. Urine analysis revealed 30 mg/dl of proteinuria and liver function tests were normal. Full blood count showed a haemoglobin 10 g/dl, haematocrit 0.35, white cell count 14×10^9/l, platelet count 180×10^9/l and a normal coagulation screen.

Placental Doppler investigation indicated that the umbilical artery end-diastolic flow was minimal and the decision was made to deliver the baby by urgent Caesarean section. Airway assessment suggested intubation would be straightforward; she had no facial oedema and a normal voice. She was given intravenous ranitidine and oral sodium citrate 30 ml for antacid prophylaxis. After discussion with the senior obstetrician and the patient, spinal anaesthesia was administered in the sitting position using 0.5% hyperbaric bupivacaine 2.5 ml and morphine 100 μg after an intravenous preload of Ringer's lactate 500 ml. This produced a bilateral anaesthetic block from T4 to S5. All observations were stable throughout, no ephedrine was required and blood loss was approximately 250 ml. After cord clamping, oxytocin 5 units was given over 5 min. A baby girl weighing 1.8 kg was delivered with Apgar scores of 8 at 5 and 10 min, and was transferred to the special care baby unit.

Postoperatively, the management was guided by the local pre-eclampsia protocol on the obstetric high dependency unit (HDU). Ringer's lactate was infused at 85 ml/h.

Four hours later, the patient complained of a headache and blurred vision, became hyper reflexic with clonus, and dropped her urine output to less than 0.5 ml/kg/h. Indirect arterial blood pressure at this time was 200/120 mmHg. Direct intra-arterial blood pressure monitoring was started and a repeat plasma profile was taken prior to central venous line insertion. Magnesium sulphate 4 g was given intravenously over 10 min followed by a continuous infusion of 1 g/h. An intravenous hydralazine infusion was started to control her persisting hypertension of 180/115 mmHg. Her platelet count had fallen to 95 $\times$ 10^9/l but coagulation remained normal. Her biochemistry was: urea 8.0 mmol/l, creatinine 110 μmol/l, uric acid 0.42 mmol/l. As the central venous pressure (CVP) was −2 mmHg, colloid 250 ml over 1 h was given. This increased the CVP to +2 mmHg and improved her urine output.

She remained stable until 16 h later, when she complained of a tight chest. She was tachypnoeic, with oxygen saturation 94% on 50% inspired oxygen. She had facial oedema, a husky voice, expiratory rhonchi and crepitations audible in both mid zones, but no stridor. A chest X-ray confirmed the presence of pulmonary oedema. The CVP had increased to +8 mmHg. Frusemide 0.5 mg/kg and nebulised salbutamol 2.5 mg were given and she was transferred to the intensive treatment unit (ITU). Her respiratory function improved with continuous positive airway pressure (CPAP) and further doses of frusemide. Electrocardiogram (ECG) and echocardiography (ECHO) were normal. Six hours later, oxygen saturation was 99% on 28% inspired oxygen via a venturi facemask, and she had diuresed 1000 ml. She returned to the obstetric HDU the next day. Magnesium and hydralazine were discontinued after 24 h and oral labetalol was started. Her subsequent recovery was uneventful.

DESCRIPTION OF THE PROBLEM

Pre-eclampsia is a multifactorial, multisystem, vascular endothelial disease of pregnancy with a variable clinical presentation. It usually occurs after 20 weeks gestation. The onset of convulsions is morphologically specific and is termed eclampsia. Eclampsia is not necessarily the end result of severe pre-eclampsia, and in many patients is not predictable using current parameters. Successive Confidential Enquiries into Maternal Deaths (CEMD) report pre-eclampsia (PIH) as the second highest cause of mortality. Common causes of death are pulmonary (respiratory distress syndrome), cerebral haemorrhage (reflecting poor hypertension control), hepatic failure or rupture and eclampsia. Fluid balance management has been highlighted as a major cause for concern.

PATHOPHYSIOLOGY

Pre-eclampsia is a disease caused by the foeto-placental unit. Multiple factors are involved, the development of immunity to paternal antigens and primipaternity are important to the pathogenesis.

Normally in early pregnancy, trophoblast cells invade the uterine spiral arteries destroying endothelium, elastin, muscle and neurones. This transforms a high-resistance arterial system into a low-resistance, high-volume system without autonomic innervation. Only endothelium is replaced, functionally identical to the old one. Endogenous vasodilators, including prostaglandin I_2 (PGI_2) and nitric oxide (NO), predominate.

In pre-eclampsia this process fails to occur in up to 50% of the spiral arteries. The endothelium is abnormal with increased permeability. Endogenous vasoconstrictors predominate with a high thromboxane A_2: prostaglandin I_2 ratio (TXA_2/PGI_2). Intense vasoconstriction causes endothelial cell damage, which together with the high levels of thromboxane A_2, result in platelet aggregation, activation of the coagulation cascade and fibrin deposition in blood vessels. Blood flow is decreased to all organs and the foeto-placental unit, resulting in ischaemia and organ dysfunction throughout the body.

Cardiovascular system

After 36 weeks gestation, Bosio *et al* using Doppler ECHO have shown a low cardiac output and high systemic vascular resistance in untreated patients. Belfort *et al* using pulmonary artery flow catheter (PAFC) in untreated patients demonstrated a low to normal cardiac output, low pulmonary capillary wedge pressure (PCWP) and high systemic vascular resistance (SVR). Benedetti *et al* have shown than a CVP greater than 6 mmHg no longer correlates with PCWP. Penny *et al* have demonstrated that Doppler ECHO underestimates the cardiac output by a mean of 36% in comparison to PAFC.

Oxygen extraction is relatively fixed, and oxygen consumption is dependent on oxygen delivery. Total blood volume is decreased by up to 40% depending on disease severity, although central blood volume is usually normal. Peripheral venous capacitance is decreased; probably due to splanchnic venoconstriction.

Interstitial oedema in the periphery and the lungs develops more easily in pre-eclampsia, especially post-partum as Starling forces across the capillary are altered.

Hydrostatic pressure is increased due to systemic hypertension, and in some patients there is left ventricular dysfunction. Hypoalbuminaemia results in a low colloid oncotic pressure (COP), reduced further after delivery as fluid shifts from the extravascular into the intravascular compartment, and with infusions of large volumes of crystalloid. Capillary permeability is increased due to abnormal endothelium. *This is why the post partum patient goes into pulmonary oedema so easily.*

Autonomic nervous system

In pre-eclampsia, around 50% of the spiral arteries retain their alpha 1 receptors and autonomic innervation, and sympathetic nerve activity is three times greater than that in normal pregnancy. There is an increased response to direct and indirect sympathetic agonists.

Renal system

The endothelial cells of the glomerulus become oedamatous with intraluminal fibrin deposition, causing a decrease in blood flow, glomerular filtration rate and the clearance of molecules. There is increased non-selective protein permeability, which quantitatively correlates with disease severity. Plasma uric acid concentration is a good indicator of disease severity as renal clearance is decreased. Pre-eclampsia rarely affects the tubules directly, with tubular ischaemia being secondary to hypovolaemia.

Hepatic system

Fibrin deposition in the sinusoids causes obstruction of blood flow from the portal into the hepatic venous systems and from the hepatic artery, which leads to oedema, haemorrhage, ischaemia and necrosis. Cell damage produces a rise in plasma aspartate aminotransferase, alanine aminotransferase and alpha–glutamyltransferase. Hepatic dysfunction is variable with decreased synthesis of coagulation factors; decreased metabolism and elimination of drugs, hormones and endotoxins; decreased blood storage; and decreased carbohydrates, protein and lipid metabolism.

The liver capsule distends resulting in epigastric and right upper quadrant pain and tenderness. Intrahepatic haemorrhage may be deep or sub-capsular, which may rupture into the peritoneal cavity.

Central nervous system

Hypertension above the normal cerebral autoregulation pressure causes increased cerebral blood flow with a high risk of intracranial haemorrhage. Disruption of the capillary blood brain barrier causes interstitial oedema.

The primary pathophysiology of eclampsia is vasospasm with secondary ischaemia and oedema. Brain tissues in the boundary zones between territories supplied by

different arteries (e.g. occipitoparietal cortex, frontal cortex, cerebellum, basal gan-
glia and brainstem) are the most vulnerable.

Haematological system

Generally, the degree of abnormality of platelets and coagulation reflect the severity
of pre-eclampsia. Disseminated intravascular coagulation is rare unless there is placental abruption. Coagulation abnormalities without placental abruption or major
haemorrhage are usually due to hepatic dysfunction.

- Platelet number and function are decreased due to microcirculatory damage, increased adhesion and aggregation.

- Decreased antithrombin III.

- Decreased blood clot strength below a platelet count of $75 \times 10^9/L$ can
  be demonstrated using thromboelastography (TEG).

- Coagulation can be considered normal above a platelet count of
  $100 \times 10^9/L$.

- Bleeding time does not correlate with platelet count or TEG with high
  inter-individual variation and poor reproducability.

MANAGEMENT OPTIONS AND DISCUSSION

Diagnosis of pre-eclampsia

Pre-eclampsia is diagnosed on the following criteria: systolic pressure >140 mmHg,
diastolic pressure >90 mmHg repeated at 6 h, and proteinuria of 30 mg/dl in a ran-
dom urine sample or >300 mg in a 24 h urine sample. It must be differentiated from
secondary non-gestational causes of hypertension occurring before 20 weeks gestation. Gestational hypertension occurring after 20 weeks gestation consists solely of
hypertension, but may be difficult to differentiate from pre-eclampsia in some patients.
Up to 25% of patients with chronic hypertension have superimposed pre-eclampsia.

Systemic blood pressure measurement

The most accurate method is by direct arterial measurement. Indirect methods of
measurement using automatic monitors based on oscillometry and Korotkoff auscultation significantly underestimate diastolic, mean and systolic pressures because
their algorithms are based on a normal population. Manual sphygmomanometry
is more accurate. Diastolic end point should be the disappearance of sound (K5)
which correlates closely to the direct diastolic pressure.

Management of acute systemic hypertension

Loss of cerebral blood flow autoregulation occurs at a mean arterial pressure of
>140 mmHg, equivalent to a BP of 180/120 mmHg, and carries a high risk of

Table 16.1 – Drugs used for the management of hypertension in pre-eclampsia. The side effects mimic impending eclampsia.

Drug	Action	Onset of action	Regimen	Side effects + Comments
Hydralazine	Direct arterial vasodilator	20 min	5 mg every 20 min or infusion	Maternal 1st line drug tachycardia, headache, nausea, vomiting
Labetalol	Non selective $\alpha + \beta$ antagonist	5 min	5–10 mg intravenously every 5 min up to a total dose of 1 mg/kg	Individual varability in β blockade 1:3 to 1:7 Foetal bradycardia
Nifedipine	Calcium antagonist	10–20 min	10 mg oral or 5 mg sublingual	Severe hypotension headache, sedation
Magnesium sulphate	Direct vasodilator and inhibitor of catecholamine release	2 min	4 g bolus. Infusion of 1–3 g/h	See below
Sodium nitroprusside	Direct arterial and venous vasodilator	4 min	Infusion of 0.05–0.1 µg/kg/min	Severe hypotension, headache, nausea, vomiting, restlessness. Foetal cyanide toxicity not a risk.

intracranial haemorrhage. Autoregulation in all organs is affected with a risk of visceral haemorrhage and rupture of thoracic and abdominal structures, ischaemia and retroplacental haemorrhage. A diastolic pressure >110 mmHg should be treated as an acute emergency guided by direct arterial monitoring, aiming for a diastolic pressure <95 mmHg while maternal organ function and foetal state should be monitored. The aim is to maintain blood pressure within maternal autoregulatory limits and protect foeto-placental blood flow as the extent of placental autoregulation is unknown. Drugs used in the acute management of hypertension are summarised in Table 16.1. Patients may already be receiving oral methyldopa or labetalol, and the total daily dose indicates disease severity.

Fluid management

The management of fluid administration differs between the ante-partum and post-partum periods (see fluid management algorithm p. 138).

Antihypertensive treatment

Antepartum, a colloid preload is given before starting treatment if the MAP <140 mm Hg as this decreases the incidence of hypotension, acute renal failure and total hypoxia. If the MAP is >140 mmHg a colloid preload is given after starting treatment.

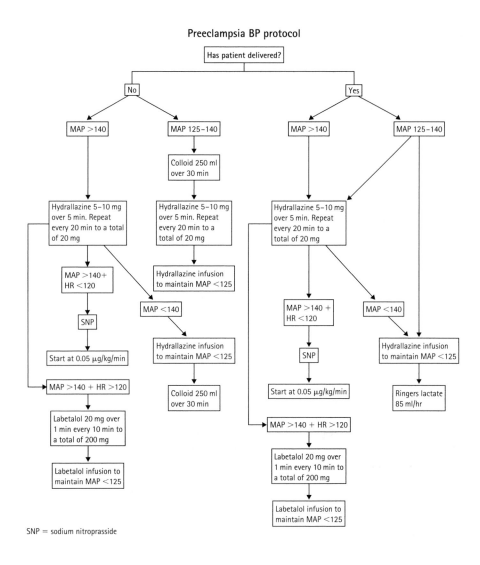

Preeclampsia BP protocol

SNP = sodium nitroprasside

Note: *Postpartum, no fluid preload is given as this increases the incidence of pulmonary oedema.*

Regional anaesthesia/analgesia

For spinal anaesthesia, preloading with 500 ml of colloid or crystalloid increases the CVP by 4 mmHg and reduces hypotension. Larger volumes increases the incidence of postpartum pulmonary oedema.

For epidural anaesthesia, preloading with 500–750 ml of Ringer's lactate decreases the incidence of hypotension.

Oliguria

Persistent oliguria is an indication for CVP monitoring. Robson measures the CVP in all patients. If the CVP is <4 mmHg a colloid preload is given, whereas if the CVP is >4 mmHg no fluid preload is given, as CVP increases greater than 10 mmHg can precipitate pulmonary oedema. If oliguria persists then liaison with the nephrologists is important.

Haemorrhage

Haemorrhage, revealed or concealed, may be due to retroplacental haemorrhage or visceral rupture. It is an acute emergency, with a high morbidity and mortality, as pre-eclamptic patients haemorrhage torrentially due to hypertension and decreased haemostasis. Haematology advice and close liaison with the blood bank are essential. Acute losses must be replaced promptly to decrease the risk of acute tubular necrosis, multiorgan ischaemia and foetal hypoxia. If the patient is ante-partum the decision to deliver the baby must be made rapidly.

Pulmonary oedema

Pulmonary oedema is a major cause of morbidity and mortality, and usually occurs post-partum. It may initially present with difficulty in breathing, an increase in respiratory rate and hypoxaemia. Decreased pulmonary compliance and increased pulmonary resistance cause increased respiratory workload. Patients in pulmonary oedema usually have iatrogenic fluid overload, acute renal failure or reduced left ventricular function. Patients should be managed on the ITU with ventilatory, renal and circulatory support, guided by advanced cardiovascular monitoring (PAFC). Some patients in pulmonary oedema may respond rapidly to frusemide and increased inspired oxygen.

The upper airway

Upper airway oedema can occur rapidly without warning signs and may present for the first time after extubation. Face, neck and tongue oedema, and voice changes are warning signs. Stridor is very rare and often occurs due to a concurrent upper respiratory tract infection. Pre-operatively, clinical laryngeal oedema can be assessed using fibreoptic nasendoscopy. Perioperatively assessment can be carried out while the patient is still anaesthetised by direct laryngoscopy.

Upper airway oedema may also occur as labour progresses, due to increases in CVP of up to 6 cmH$_2$O with each contraction and up to 50 cmH$_2$O in the second stage. This can be modified by epidural analgesia.

Oedematous tissue has decreased compliance so that it is more difficult to move the hyoid bone forward and downward in order to elevate the epiglottis, and visualise the larynx. If the neck is oedematous, the identification of the cricoid cartilage and cricothyroid membrane is more difficult.

Table 16.2 – Management of eclampsia.

- ABC resuscitation.
- Magnesium 4 g over 5–10 min + maintenance infusion starting at 1–2 g/h

For recurrent convulsions while receiving magnesium:

- Administer magnesium 2 g if < 70 kg, 4 g if > 70 kg over 5 min and consider diazepam 2.5 mg
- Consider airway protection and ventilation to decrease the risk of pulmonary aspiration
- Pharmacological and physiological control of ↑ ICP.
- Consider CT scan and neurosurgical opinion.

Acute renal failure

Oliguria <0.5 ml/kg/h for two consecutive hours is common immediately before delivery and for 12–18 h post-partum. Uncorrected hypovolaemia decreases placental blood flow and increases the risk of acute renal failure.

Acute renal failure is a rare complication of well-managed pre-eclampsia and is associated with post-partum haemorrhage and placental abruption. The cause is acute tubular necrosis (medullary necrosis), which is usually reversible and recovers within 6 weeks. When other predisposing conditions are present, the pathology is cortical necrosis, acute renal failure is more likely to be irreversible.

Eclampsia

Impending eclampsia can present with headache, vomiting, cerebral hyper-reactivity (hyper-reflexia, clonus, jitteriness), visual disturbances, acute confusion, pyramidal motor dysfunction, extrapyramidal motor dysfunction, central somatic sensory dysfunction and acute psychosis. The treatment is summarised in Table 16.2.

The differential diagnosis of any convulsion is essential, especially where there has been no previous diagnosis of pre-eclampsia. Neurological examination for focal signs of intracranial haemorrhage should be carried out with radiological and neurosurgical management as appropriate. Multiple pathologies must be thought of, if an eclamptic patient is not responding to management. Eclampsia may occur up to 23 days after delivery.

Convulsion prophylaxis

Although magnesium is known to be effective in preventing further fits in eclampsia, its use as prophylaxis in pre-eclampsia has until recently been controversial. However, the recently published Magpie trial showed that magnesium is effective in reducing the progression to eclampsia and is safe to mother and baby.

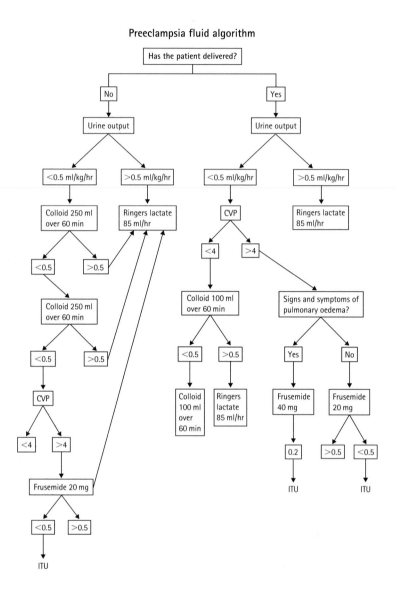

Preeclampsia fluid algorithm

Magnesium

The main mechanism of action of magnesium is by antagonism of calcium and decreasing synaptic transmission. Ischaemia causes a reduction in the transmembrane potential and increases calcium transport into the cell, resulting in mitochondrial dysfunction and oedema. Magnesium antagonises this by inhibiting calcium transport via the voltage-gated N-methyl-D-aspartate (NMDA) channel. Magnesium also decreases cerebral and retinal vasospasm, and is specific for convulsions due to eclampsia.

Table 16.3 – Signs and symptoms associated with different plasma magnesium concentrations.

Magnesium blood concentration	Effect
0.7–1.1 mmol/l	Normal
2–3.5 mmol/l	Therapeutic
4–6.5 mmol/l	Nausea and vomiting, drowsiness, double vision, slurring of speech and loss of tendon reflexes
6.5–7.5 mmol/l	Muscle paralysis and respiratory arrest
>10 mmol/l	Cardiac arrest in diastole

Magnesium is a direct vasodilator and decreases catecholamine release from the adrenal medulla and adrenergic neurones. It decreases calcium entry into myocardial cells, decreasing sinoatrial (SA) and atrioventricular (AV) node conduction, and increasing the AV node refractory period. Overall, CVS effects are decreased systemic and pulmonary vascular resistance (SVR and PVR) and systemic BP with a secondary increase in myocardial contractility and cardiac output. It is anti-arrhythmic.

At the neuromuscular junction, magnesium reduces presynaptic acetylcholine release and it decreases the sensitivity of the postsynaptic membrane to acetylcholine, causing a decrease in membrane excitability. This results in neuromuscular junction blockade. Magnesium increases the duration of action of non-depolarising neuromuscular junction blocking drugs and fasciculations after suxamethonium are significantly decreased.

Magnesium increases PGI_2 release which decreases platelet adhesion and aggregation. James *et al*, using TEG, demonstrated no effect on clot strength below 5 mmol/l.

Magnesium crosses the placenta and decreases foetal heart rate variability, which may make interpretation difficult. It also decreases uterine myometrial contractility. Although there is no statistically significant increase in haemorrhage, there is an increase in oxytocin requirement.

Monitoring magnesium concentration

Magnesium therapy is safe if the patient is appropriately monitored according to a local protocol and careful attention is taken of urine output, as magnesium is 100% eliminated renally. Safe administration of magnesium requires regular monitoring of urine output, respiratory rate and tendon reflexes to detect early toxicity (see Table 16.3). Clinical monitoring can be supplemented by serum magnesium levels. Emergency management of overdose consists of ABC resuscitation and calcium glutamate 10% over 10 min.

Planning delivery of the foetus

The timing of delivery is a multidisciplinary decision. The patient should be stabilised before delivery *especially if* eclampsia has occurred. Monitoring for maternal and foetal complications should be continuous, and trends in all parameters are more important than a single reading or result. The most important parameter in the determination of foetal outcome is the gestational age. To improve foetal pulmonary maturity, prophylactic steroids should be administered to patients less than 34 weeks gestation and before 32 weeks gestation, Caesarean section should be considered.

Regional anaesthesia

A normal coagulation profile and a platelet count $>80 \times 10^9/l$ (within 2 h) are generally required before considering regional anaesthesia. Although theoretically, spinal anaesthesia should produce greater haemodynamic instability than epidural anaesthesia, in practice, there is little difference in the incidence of hypotension and spinal anaesthesia produces superior anaesthesia.

Lumbar epidural analgesia during labour decreases central and peripheral sympathetic and endocrine output. The resulting decreases in SVR and heart rate attenuate the large rises in BP and CVP that occur during labour.

Infusions of bupivacaine 0.1% with fentanyl 2 µg/ml result in improved haemodynamic stability and organ perfusion compared with intermittent local anaesthetic bolus techniques. The addition of *vasoconstrictors* to local anaesthetic solutions is best avoided. The dose of vasopressors should be reduced.

General anaesthesia

Pre-operatively, careful airway assessment and identification of the cricothyroid membrane should be carried out. Blood investigations should be repeated within 2 h as rapid deterioration may occur. Haematological advice should be requested as appropriate and blood products, if required, should be ordered and ready in theatre before starting surgery. The following problems should be considered:

- *Difficult intubation and pre-operative laryngeal oedema* Difficult airway management equipment should be to hand, including a short-handled laryngoscope, a range of smaller diameter tracheal tubes, a fibreoptic bronchoscope, and equipment for cricothyrotomy and transtracheal jet ventilation. Pre-operative stridor from laryngeal oedema is rare, and should be treated with nebulised epinephrine 5 mg and dexamethasone 0.2 mg/kg. Nasendoscopic assessment of the larynx under local anaesthesia and senior ENT surgical advice help determine optimum management of the airway. Laryngeal oedema not severe enough to cause signs and symptoms pre-operatively, but present at laryngoscopy, will require a smaller diameter tracheal tube. Laryngeal oedema may occur for the first time after extubation, and should be checked for whilst the patient is still anaesthetised.

- *Increased sympathetic response to intubation and extubation* The sympathetic and endocrine response to intubation requires attenuation as there is a high risk of intracranial haemorrhage, myocardial ischaemia, cardiac arrhythmias, pulmonary oedema and foetal hypoxia. Pre-induction administration of magnesium 60 mg/kg, if the patient is not on magnesium and 40 mg/kg if the patient is, has been suggested by Allen *et al.* It should be administered approximately 90 seconds preintubation. Magnesium seems to be the ideal agent, as it does not cause foetal respiratory depression (opioids), foetal hypoglycaemia or precipitous maternal hypotension (hydrallazine SNP).

- *Neuromuscular blocking agents' onset and duration* Plasma cholinesterase levels are decreased by up to 30% in pre-eclampsia, so the duration of action of suxamethonium is increased. The duration of non-depolarising neuromuscular blocking drugs is increased. As fasciculations after suxamethonium are significantly reduced, a peripheral nerve stimulator should be used to assess optimum time for intubation.

Other drugs

Oxytocin should be given slowly as it causes systemic vasodilatation and pulmonary vasoconstriction. Ergometrine should be avoided as it causes vasoconstriction and may precipitate eclampsia. Non-steroidal anti-inflammatory drugs should be avoided if there is significant intra-operative haemorrhage, thrombocytopaenia, coagulopathy, oliguria or renal dysfunction.

Postoperative management

A spontaneous diuresis is an important sign that the patient is improving. The patient should remain on HDU/ITU until all parameters normalise.

KEY LEARNING POINTS

1. Early and effective interdisciplinary communication and teamwork is important.

2. There should be local obstetric unit guidelines.

3. A system for the safe, rapid interhospital transfer of patients should be in place.

4. Overall responsibility and particularly fluid management for each patient should be by one clinician.

5. Management of all patients with severe pre-eclampsia should be on a HDU.

6. Fluid management depends upon whether the patient is antepartum or post-partum.

7. CVP should be maintained below 4 mmHg.

8. Rapid deterioration of clinical and plasma parameters may occur. Trends in these parameters are more important than absolute values.

9. The prophylactic management of multiorgan failure may be a way forward for the future as mortality from this is high.

Further reading

Allen RW, James MFM, Uys PC. Attenuation of the pressor response to tracheal intubation in hypertensive proteinuric pregnant patients by lignocaine, alfentanil and magnesium sulphate. *British Journal of Anaesthesia* 1991; **66**: 216–23.

Belfort MA, Anthony J, Saade GR *et al.* The oxygen consumption/oxygen delivery curve in severe pre-eclampsia: evidence for a fixed oxygen extraction. *American Journal of Obstetrics and Gynecology* 1993; **169**: 1448–55.

Bosio PM, McKenna PJ, Conroy R *et al.* Maternal central haemodynamics in hypertensive disorders of pregnancy. *Obstetrics and Gynaecology* 1999; **94**: 978–84.

Coetzee EJ, Dommisse J, Anthony J. A randomised controlled trial of intravenous magnesium sulphate versus placebo in the management of women with severe pre eclampsia. *British Journal of Obstetrics and Gynaecology* 1998; **105**: 300–303.

Dekker GA, Sibai BM. Etiology and pathogenesis of pre-eclampsia: current concepts. *American Journal of Obstetrics and Gynecology* 1998; **179**: 1359–75.

Douglas KA, Redman CWG. Eclampsia in the United Kingdom. *British Medical Journal* 1994; **309**: 1395–400.

Higgins JR, de Swiet M. Blood pressure measurement and classification in pregnancy. *Lancet* 2001; **357**: 131–5.

James MFM, Neil G. Effect of magnesium on coagulation as measured by thrombelastography. *British Journal of Anaesthesia* 1995; **74**: 92–4.

Katz VL, Farmer R, Kuller JA. Preeclampsia into eclampsia: toward a new paradigm. *American Journal of Obstetrics and Gynecology* 2000; **182**: 1389–98.

Natarajan P, Shennan AH, Penny J et al. Comparison of auscultatory and oscillo-metric automated blood pressure monitors in the setting of pre-eclampsia. *American Journal of Obstetrics and Gynecology* 1999; **181**: 1203–10.

Naidu K, Moodley J, Corr P et al. Single photon emission and cerebral comput-erised tomographic scan and transcranial Doppler sonographic findings in eclampsia. *British Journal of Obstetrics and Gynaecology* 1997; **104**: 1165–72.

The Magpie Trial Collaboration Group. Do women with pre-eclampsia, and their babies, benefit from magnesium sulphate? The Magpie trial: a randomised placebo-controlled trial. *Lancet* 2002; **359**: 1877–90.

Penny JA, Anthony J, Shennan AH, *et al.* A comparison of pulmonary artery flota-tion catheter and the oesophageal Doppler monitor in pre eclampsia. *American Journal of Obstetrics and Gynecology* 2000; **183**: 658–61.

Ramanathan J, Sibai BM, Pillai R, Angel JJ. Neuromuscular transmission studies in preeclamptic women receiving magnesium sulphate. *American Journal of Obstetrics and Gynecology* 1998; **158**: 40–6.

Robson SC. Fluid restriction policies in pre eclampsia are obsolete. *International Journal of Obstetric Anesthesia* 1999; **8**: 49–55.

Sharma SK, Philip J, Whitten CW, *et al.* Assessment of changes in coagulation in parturients with pre eclampsia using thromboelastography. *Anesthesiology* 1999; **90**: 385–90.

Sharwood-Smith G, Clark V, Watson E. Regional anaesthesia for caesarean section in severe pre eclampsia: spinal anaesthesia is the preferred choice. *International Journal of Obstetric Anesthesia* 1999; **8**: 85–9.

Silver HM, Seebeck M, Carlson R. Comparison of total blood volume in normal, preeclamptic, and non-proteinuric gestational hypertensive pregnancy by simultaneous measurement of red blood cell and plasma volumes. *American Journal of Obstetrics and Gynecology* 1998; **179**: 87–93.

17

SPINAL SURGERY AND THE OBSTETRIC PATIENT

S.K. Krishnan and C.C. Callander

CASE HISTORY

A 33-year-old female was referred to the anaesthetic assessment clinic in the 24th week of pregnancy. Her two previous pregnancies, 8 and 5 years before, had resulted in spontaneous vaginal deliveries. The latter delivery included epidural analgesia. Four years prior to the current pregnancy, she developed symptoms and signs of lumbar disc prolapse and underwent a partial L5/S1 laminectomy and discectomy. Following surgery, her back pain settled and she was left with only occasional, minor radicular pain in her right leg. During this pregnancy, her back pain became worse with occasional pain radiating to the right hip and medial aspect of the foot.

At the anaesthetic assessment clinic she wished to discuss epidural analgesia. She had unpleasant memories of pain with her first delivery and was keen to repeat her experience of her second delivery and have an epidural. She was, however, concerned about any long-term effects from the epidural on her pre-existing back problem.

On examination, she was 160 cm tall and weighed 62 kg. She had a surgical scar over her lumbar spine extending from approximately L4 to the sacrum. There was tenderness over the L4/5 interspace. Neurological examination did not reveal any abnormality.

It was explained to her that regional analgesia should still be possible, but that there could be some difficulty with insertion and the resultant analgesia might be patchy. She was reassured that the epidural should not cause any long-term problems with her back. Following this discussion, she opted to wait and see how her labour pains developed before deciding, but she was glad to know that an epidural would probably be possible. A final point she

---

raised was whether or not she should have an elective Caesarean section to 'protect her back'. She was advised to discuss this with her obstetrician but the point was made that regional anaesthesia would certainly be open to her.

At term, she was admitted in early labour. She requested an epidural after vaginal examination showed her cervix to be 4 cm dilated. An epidural catheter was inserted at the L1/2 interspace. There was no difficulty in identifying the space nor was there any paraesthesia during epidural insertion. A test dose of 3 ml bupivacaine 0.5% was followed by 10 ml bupivacaine 0.25% with fentanyl 5 µg/ml. The upper level of analgesia was T7 bilaterally but the block did not extend below L4 on the right side. A further 10 ml bupivacaine 0.1% was administered in the right lateral decubitus position. After 10 min, the uterine contractions were painfree. An infusion of 12 ml/h bupivacaine 0.1% with fentanyl 3 µg/ml was then commenced. Further boluses of 10 ml bupivacaine 0.25% were required at 2 and 4 h due to breakthrough pain from an insufficient block of the lower right lumbar and sacral roots. After 7 h, a Caesarean section was necessary for failure to progress. In view of the recurring problems of inadequate epidural analgesia, we decided to administer a subarachnoid block using 2.5 ml hyperbaric bupivacaine 0.5% and 100 µg preservative-free morphine, administered in the sitting position via a 27 g pencil tip needle inserted at the L3/4 interspace. Care was taken to avoid a high block by initially placing the patient in a slightly head up position. Anaesthesia from T4 to S5 bilaterally was achieved. An uneventful Caesarean section and recovery then followed. There was no post-partum exacerbation of the pre-existing back problem.

DESCRIPTION OF THE PROBLEM

The provision of regional analgesia and anaesthesia in a parturient with a history of spinal surgery requires careful consideration of several factors.

1. There may be technical difficulty in identifying the epidural space.

2. The spread of local anaesthetic solution may be uneven leading to patchy analgesia.

3. The patient may be concerned about an exacerbation of back pain in the post-partum period.

This chapter focuses on the issues associated with surgery for lumbar disc prolapse. Major spinal surgery for kyphoscoliosis raises other, separate issues and is discussed elsewhere.

PATHOPHYSIOLOGY

Abnormal vertebral anatomy is associated with a significant epidural failure rate and an increase in the risk of accidental dural puncture. The technical difficulty associated with epidural placement in patients who have a history of lumbar spine surgery has been prospectively investigated in 1381 patients undergoing epidural anaesthesia for total hip or knee replacement surgery (see Sharrock *et al.* in further reading). Patients who had a past history of lumbar spine surgery had a 91.2% rate of successful epidural placement (52 out of 57 cases). Patients without previous surgery had a 98.7% rate of successful epidural placement (1307 out of 1324 cases, $P < 0.0001$). The authors also addressed the question of inadvertent dural puncture. Postoperatively, the dura may become tethered to the ligamentum flavum by scar tissue. They recommended that the optimal site of epidural insertion should be one, or preferably two, interspaces above the surgical scar. There are no similar studies on large numbers of parturients but there are individual case reports relating to previous spinal surgery, which show that altered spread of local anaesthetic in the epidural space can occur. The possible causes include epidural adhesions, fibrous bands and tethering of dura mater. Ineffective spread has been confirmed in radiological studies of the epidural space. Typically, there is sacral sparing, but this may be only unilateral. Increased cephalad spread may occur due to the physical barrier limiting lower movement of local anaesthetic in the epidural space. Availability of previous X-rays, MRI studies and possibly ultrasonography can be of great help in drawing up management plans.

MANAGEMENT OPTIONS (AND DISCUSSION)

Uneven analgesia

Various measures to overcome the problem of unblocked segments have been suggested. Larger volumes of more concentrated local anaesthetic combined with vasopressor drugs and/or opioids have been used. In theory, a second epidural catheter can be inserted below the supposed obstruction, but in practice, this is not usually feasible due to the presence of scar tissue. A caudal epidural would bypass the surgical site and should produce effective sacral blockade, but in most centres this is not a commonly used procedure in labouring women. One final option is intrathecal analgesia. A single-shot intrathecal injection would provide effective analgesia but of limited duration. This is usually possible and useful for severe pain in late labour. An intrathecal catheter allows the delivery of prolonged analgesia and has been described in a scoliosis patient where an epidural failed.

In our case history, the epidural was placed two spaces above the surgical scar as recommended. There are no studies showing this to be essential but it would seem to be advisable so as to minimise the risk of accidental dural puncture in a patient with a disrupted epidural space. The epidural catheter was introduced without any technical problems, but the resultant block was patchy. Unblocked segments during continuous lumbar epidural analgesia can occur in normal patients; however, reports suggest that spinal surgery patients are at a small, but significantly greater risk of this problem. We elected to use an intrathecal technique when Caesarean section became necessary in view of the limited spread of the epidural analgesia. A good intrathecal block can be achieved in cases where physical barriers to epidural spread are present. Caution is required when superimposing intrathecal anaesthesia on partially-effective epidural analgesia. The 'filled' epidural space may cause the dura to be slightly compressed resulting in an unpredictable high level of spinal block. Smaller doses of intrathecal local anaesthetic or judicious patient positioning are advised. For elective Caesarean section, a standard intrathecal technique is appropriate.

Concerns of worsening back pain

Our patient was particularly concerned about the possibility of long-term effects from an epidural on her pre-existing back problem. Back pain in the post-partum period has been reported in 30–45% of women receiving epidural analgesia. Retrospective surveys have found an association between epidural analgesia and back pain but no causal link. More recently, however, several prospective surveys have failed to find any significant difference between women who received epidural analgesia and those who did not. Any back pain related to epidural analgesia appears to be restricted to the first post-partum week. Among all demographic, obstetric and epidural variables examined, only a previous history of back pain is significantly associated with post-partum back pain. Patients who have back pain during their pregnancy are at increased risk of developing post-partum back pain, whether or not the back pain had existed before pregnancy. Patients with only a history of back pain before pregnancy and not during pregnancy appear not to have an increased risk of developing post-partum pain. The patient in our case report did have significant problems with her back during the pregnancy and she was advised that she would probably have further back trouble after delivery and that there might be an exacerbation of her symptoms. She was reassured, however, that having an epidural would not increase her risk of worsening back trouble.

Planning for delivery

The benefits of seeing such patients in anaesthetic pre-assessment clinics cannot be overstated. It is highly unsatisfactory to first encounter these patients in the middle of the night when they are in established labour and have already received opioids and Entonox, making it difficult to have a meaningful discussion about the risks and benefits of epidural analgesia. Furthermore, it is unlikely that there will be time to obtain casenotes and essential old X-rays relating to previous back surgery. Back pain with or without surgery can have a dramatic impact on quality of life and the fear of exacerbation can dominate the patient's thoughts. Their worries about the pain they may suffer from their back during labour can lead to extreme anxiety throughout pregnancy and may even over ride any positive thoughts about their baby. In this context, it is immensely beneficial to be able to reassure patients that good epidural analgesia probably can be provided in labour and that this will not have a detrimental effect on their long-term back problems. It is striking how such patients welcome the chance to discuss their concerns. They often use the opportunity to raise issues such as the option of elective Caesarean section to 'protect their back' from the impact of a long labour. Issues such as these can then be addressed in the cold light of day well in advance of the delivery date. Fully discussing risks and benefits, and involving these patients in drawing up management plans is particularly necessary in order to achieve the highest maternal satisfaction.

KEY LEARNING POINTS

1. Parturients who have a history of lumbar disc surgery benefit greatly from assessment and advice at an anaesthetic assessment clinic.

2. Epidural analgesia is usually possible, but there is a slightly higher failure rate than in the normal population.

3. Patients should be reassured that epidural techniques should not worsen their underlying back problem.

4. Intrathecal techniques should be successful even if there has been difficulty with an epidural.

Further reading

Breen TW, Ransil BJ, Groves P, Oriol NE. Factors associated with back pain after childbirth. *Anesthesiology* 1994; **81**: 29–34.

Calleja MA. Extradural analgesia and previous spinal surgery. *Anaesthesia* 1991; **46**: 946-7.

MacArthur C, Lewis M, Knox EG, Crawford JS. Epidural anaesthesia and long term backache after childbirth. *British Medical Journal* 1990; **301**: 9–12.

Moran DH, Johnson MD. Continuous spinal anaesthesia with combined hyperbaric and isobaric bupivacaine in a patient with scoliosis. *Anesthesia and Analgesia* 1990; **70**: 445–7.

Pascoe HF, Jennings SG, Marx GF. Successful spinal anesthesia after inadequate epidural block in a parturient with prior surgical correction of scoliosis. *Regional Anesthesia* 1993; **18**: 191–2.

Robinson PN, Salmon P, Yentis SM. Maternal satisfaction. *International Journal of Obstetric Anesthesia* 1998; **7**: 32–7.

Russell R, Dundas R, Reynolds F. Long term backache after childbirth: prospective search for causative factors. *British Medical Journal* 1996; **312**: 1384–8.

Schachner SA, Abram SE. Use of two epidural catheters to provide analgesia of unblocked segments in a patient with lumbar disc disease. *Anesthesiology* 1982; **56**: 150–1.

Sharrock NE, Urquhart B, Mineo R. Extradural anaesthesia in patients with previous lumbar spine surgery. *British Journal of Anaesthesia* 1990; **65**: 237–9.

18

SUXAMETHONIUM APNOEA IN PREGNANCY

J.S.S. Davies

CASE HISTORY

A 28-year-old, gravida 2, para 1, woman was referred to a consultant obstetric anaesthetist at 23 weeks gestation because she had been noted at booking to carry a 'Medi-Alert' tag on which was written 'allergic to scoline'. Her height was 1.60 m and weight 90.6 kg (body mass index $= 35\,kg/m^2$). Her first pregnancy, 6 years previously, ended with a spontaneous vaginal delivery and she received Entonox and pethidine for analgesia.

The patient had no further documentation to explain her condition and had never received a general anaesthetic. However, she had a clear recollection of having a blood test as a child after a sibling had problems under general anaesthesia. She was subsequently told that the reaction to the drug was 'inherited and left affected people paralysed'. On this evidence, it was assumed that the patient was either heterozygous or homozygous for one of the varieties of abnormal plasma cholinesterase. We decided that further cholinesterase analysis at this stage would not be helpful due to the misleading effects of pregnancy. There was sufficient evidence to avoid the use of suxamethonium in any necessary anaesthetic intervention, using regional anaesthesia where possible, and encouraging epidural analgesia for labour. Clinical assessments of the patient's neck and jaw movements were performed which suggested that tracheal intubation would be straightforward. The potential problems of anaesthetic management were explained to the patient and documented in her notes. She was advised to ensure that the anaesthetist was informed when she was admitted in labour.

The patient was next seen by an anaesthetist soon after her admission at 39 weeks gestation with spontaneous onset of labour. Cervical dilatation was noted to be 4–5 cm on initial vaginal examination and preparations were made for insertion of an epidural catheter as planned. At this point, the patient became significantly more distressed and the foetal heart monitor showed persistent late foetal heart rate decelerations. The midwife contacted the obstetrician who examined the patient again and found the cervix dilated to 6 cm and, therefore decided to proceed to emergency Caesarean section.

The patient already had an intravenous infusion in progress, appropriate monitoring was attached and the patient placed in a right lateral position for attempted insertion of a combined spinal–epidural (CSE) by a needle-through-needle technique. This was considered to offer the best compromise of rapid speed of onset and confidence in establishing a good block, thus avoiding the need for general anaesthesia. Following the intrathecal injection of 2.5 ml hyperbaric bupivacaine 0.5% with preservative-free morphine 100 µg, the epidural catheter was successfully passed and secured. The patient was then placed in a supine position with left tilt. At 5 min, the patient was found to have a good block, with anaesthesia to light touch up to and including T4 bilaterally. The Caesarean section was commenced and proceeded uneventfully, and a live male infant with Apgar scores of 8 and 10 was delivered.

DEFINITION OF THE PROBLEM

Patients sensitive to suxamethonium due to abnormalities in their plasma cholinesterase pose a particular problem to the obstetric anaesthetist due to the importance of the drug in rapid sequence induction, the mainstay of obstetric general anaesthesia. It is vital that the anaesthetist is notified of such patients in good time so that further enquiries and investigations into the patient's status can occur, and a management plan made.

PATHOPHYSIOLOGY

Soon after the introduction of suxamethonium into clinical use in 1952, it was noticed that a small number of patients would remain paralysed and apnoeic for prolonged periods after a single dose. It was known that plasma cholinesterase was responsible for the metabolism of suxamethonium and by analysing the cholinesterase activity of samples of plasma and measuring the degree of inhibition of the reaction by certain agents, a picture of the different phenotypes was developed. This knowledge, together with the patterns found in affected families, allowed the definition of an increasing number of genotypical variations for which a particular patient could be homozygous or heterozygous. At present, the genotypes are atypical, fluoride resistant, a number of silent genes, as well as J, K and H variants. Patients homozygous for all these variations demonstrate a reduction in cholinesterase activity of between 30% below normal to no activity at all. Those who are heterozygous for these variations are likely to have much smaller reductions in their cholinesterase activity, which does not usually lead to any clinically significant effect.

Plasma cholinesterase activity is also reduced by pregnancy. The mean reduction is 24% by the end of the first trimester, which is sustained through the rest of the pregnancy; it is further reduced to 33% below normal in the first week post-partum before returning to normal values by 6 weeks post-partum. The reasons for these changes are not known. These changes alone are not sufficient to cause any demonstrable change in the duration of action of suxamethonium. However, patients who are heterozygous for one of the abnormal genes, and not normally affected may have an increased duration of action when given suxamethonium during pregnancy. It is possible, therefore, that a patient who has previously been given suxamethonium without untoward effect may exhibit a prolonged response during or immediately after pregnancy. There is also some evidence to suggest an increased likelihood of placental transfer of suxamethonium when the mother has sustained levels due to low cholinesterase activity.

MANAGEMENT OPTIONS AND DISCUSSION

Antenatal preparation

The most common indication for the use of general anaesthesia, and therefore suxamethonium, in current obstetric anaesthetic practice is the need to conduct an urgent operative delivery for the good of the foetus. The anaesthetic management of patients with proven or potential suxamethonium apnoea poses a number of interesting problems. Ideally, such problems should be contemplated beforehand. This requires those responsible for booking patients (midwives or obstetricians) to be aware of the importance of the condition, and to make arrangements for an anaesthetic opinion in the middle trimester, before the time when anaesthetic intervention is most likely. Further investigation of the patient at this stage is difficult because of the changes in cholinesterase seen in pregnancy. It may be useful in a patient with a vague history, when a normal or slightly reduced level of cholinesterase activity might provide reassurance that suxamethonium may be used safely. In a patient with a proven abnormality, however, it is best to devise a plan of action to avoid its use. Plasma cholinesterase is in fact preserved in stored blood and fresh frozen plasma, but it would be difficult to justify transfusion purely to supplement cholinesterase activity in view of the potential for transmission of infective agents.

Regional anaesthesia

In most cases, this means that regional anaesthesia should be chosen for whatever obstetric intervention that becomes necessary. This does not avoid the potential need for general anaesthesia; a small proportion of patients will need conversion to general anaesthesia either due to inability to establish a block, or due to an inadequate block causing intra-operative pain. It is, therefore, important to choose the most reliable method of regional anaesthesia and that it is performed with due care to minimise the chance of conversion.

If a patient is expected to labour, it is sensible to provide epidural analgesia early in the first stage as most anaesthetists would feel more confident topping up a good epidural than establishing a spinal when there is some urgency to deliver. It is also important to ensure that the epidural is effective. For elective Caesarean section, the method of choice is either a spinal or a CSE. A CSE is theoretically the better option as it allows the extent or duration of the block to be increased. Anaesthetists unfamiliar with the CSE technique may prefer to use a single-shot spinal injection, although in an elective situation there is sufficient time to consult with colleagues and cope with the practicalities of a CSE. Whichever method is chosen, if it proves impossible to establish an adequate block, there is always the opportunity to have another attempt on another day as a fall back position.

In an emergency or urgent situation, there remains the same choice of spinal or CSE, but now the personal experience of the anaesthetist concerned becomes a more important factor, especially in a true emergency Caesarean section.

Despite an intention to use regional anaesthesia, it is important that a plan for general anaesthesia is prepared, as there is always the potential for having to convert to general anaesthesia. In addition, there may be contraindications to regional anaesthesia, such as lack of consent, local or systemic sepsis, coagulopathy, spinal cord disease or abnormalities, and actual or potential major haemorrhage. Lack of consent for regional anaesthesia is relatively uncommon these days with greater acceptance of regional anaesthesia for Caesarean section. There is also increasing recognition that major haemorrhage is not necessarily a contraindication to regional anaesthesia.

General anaesthesia

If general anaesthesia is necessary, a decision has to be made whether to proceed with a rapid sequence induction avoiding suxamethonium, or secure the airway by an awake fibreoptic intubation prior to induction of anaesthesia. If a modified rapid sequence induction is used, rocuronium is currently the muscle relaxant of choice due to its relatively rapid onset. However, due to its much longer duration of action than suxamethonium, there would need to be a high level of confidence that intubation would be possible. Many different clinical tests predicting likely ease or difficulty in intubation exist; most importantly, the pre-operative assessment should be performed shortly before induction, even if it has been done previously, as many factors affecting intubation can change as pregnancy progresses. It is also appropriate that such an assessment and the subsequent induction are performed or directly supervised by an experienced anaesthetist. Similarly, if an awake fibreoptic intubation is planned, it should be performed by someone experienced in the technique. Oral intubation is more suitable than the nasal route because of the likelihood of nasal oedema and hyperaemia in pregnancy.

A cholinesterase abnormality may first come to light when suxamethonium is used during an obstetric general anaesthetic. Assuming that intubation is achieved, there is no reason for this being any more than an unpleasant surprise for the anaesthetist. The patient should not be at any risk, as long as a peripheral nerve stimulator is used routinely to demonstrate recovery from suxamethonium before a non-depolarising neuromuscular blocking drug is given. Our obstetric colleagues will appreciate us not waiting for clinical signs of the suxamethonium wearing off as this often coincides with them delivering the baby. In this situation, where the concentration of suxamethonium in the maternal circulation is sustained at high levels, the paediatrician should be alerted to the possibility of placental transfer of the drug.

KEY LEARNING POINTS

1. Ideally, patients with suxamethonium apnoea should be reviewed in the middle trimester so that an anaesthetic treatment plan can be formulated.

2. Regional anaesthesia should be used unless contra-indicated, and should be conducted as carefully as possible.

3. A plan for safe general anaesthesia should be made in case it is necessary.

4. One should always be aware of the possibility of discovering a previously undiagnosed case of suxamethonium apnoea during an obstetric general anaesthetic.

Further reading

Baraka A, Haroun S, Bassili M, *et al*. Response of the newborn to succinylcholine injection in homozygotic atypical mothers. *Anesthesiology* 1975; **43**: 115–16.

Broomhead CJ, Davies W, Higgins D. Awake oral fibreoptic intubation for caesarean section. *International Journal of Obstetric Anesthesia* 1995; **4**: 172–4.

Davis L, Britten JJ, Morgan M. Cholinesterase. Its significance in anaesthetic practice. *Anaesthesia* 1997; **52**: 244–60.

Parekh N, Husaini SWU, Russell IF. Caesarean section for placenta praevia: a retrospective study of anaesthetic management. *British Journal of Anaesthesia* 2000; **84**: 725–30.

Whittaker M. Plasma cholinesterase variants and the anaesthetist. *Anaesthesia* 1980; **35**: 174–97.

Whittaker M, Crawford JS, Lewis M. Some observations of levels of plasma cholinesterase activity within an obstetric population. *Anaesthesia* 1988; **43**: 42–5.

19

THROMBOCYTOPAENIA IN PREGNANCY

K.A. Eggers

CASE HISTORY

A 34-year-old Caucasian female, gravida 2, para 1, presented to the antenatal clinic at 12 weeks gestation. She weighed 82.9 kg and her body mass index (BMI) was 29 kg/m^2. Chronic idiopathic thrombocytopaenia (immune thrombocytopenic purpura, ITP) had been diagnosed during her first pregnancy and confirmed postnatally. An emergency lower-segment Caesarean section had been performed under general anaesthesia at 32 weeks gestation for worsening pre-eclampsia, complicated by ITP. She had no allergies and was taking no medications. There were no bruises or petechiae on physical examination and her blood pressure was 120/80 mmHg. Investigations included a full blood count (haemoglobin concentration 12.6 g/dl, white blood cell count 6.2×10^9/l, platelets 54×10^9/l), normal coagulation screen, her blood group was O positive, rubella antibodies were detected and alpha-foetoprotein screening was declined.

This second pregnancy continued uneventfully and the obstetricians and haematologists saw her regularly. She was referred for an obstetric anaesthetic assessment at 28 weeks. She wished to avoid regional anaesthesia and opted for a general anaesthetic if operative delivery was required. Her platelet count declined to 40×10^9/l at 30 weeks. This was treated with prednisolone 1 mg/kg/day until her platelet count stabilised at 60×10^9/l on a maintenance dose of 5 mg per day. Her blood pressure remained stable throughout this pregnancy. An ultrasound scan at 34 weeks gestation showed a single live foetus, breech presentation, posterior placenta and no praevia. In view of this, an elective lower-segment Caesarean section was planned for 38 weeks gestation. At this time, her platelet count had fallen to 35×10^9/l.

Prior to surgery, she received intravenous immunoglobulin 0.4 g/kg for 5 days in an attempt to raise the platelet count. Despite this, on the day of the delivery her platelet count was still only 45×10^9/l. Therefore, platelets were arranged to be immediately available in case of excessive bleeding. Standard premedication of oral ranitidine and sodium citrate was given. General anaesthesia was administered with regard to obstetric anaesthetic principles. No significant bleeding occurred, and crystalloid 1000 ml and colloid 500 ml were infused. She received patient-controlled anaesthesia (PCA) morphine for postoperative analgesia; diclofenac and intramuscular injections were avoided.

The baby's cord blood showed a platelet count of 104×10^9/l. Over the next 5 days, no signs of neonatal bleeding were seen. Both mother and baby were discharged home after 7 days.

DEFINITION OF THE PROBLEM

Maternal thrombocytopaenia is relatively common, usually asymptomatic and benign. Recent guidelines have been produced for the investigation and management of thrombocytopaenia in pregnancy. Appropriate assessment and investigation is important in order to identify a remedial cause and prevent unnecessary and potentially hazardous interventions for mother and foetus. Antenatal referral to the obstetric anaesthetist should occur to consider the safety of regional techniques in these patients.

PATHOPHYSIOLOGY

Thrombocytopaenia is the most common platelet disorder to affect pregnancy and may be physiological or pathological. The reduction in platelet count may be secondary to a decreased production, sequestration in the spleen or, more commonly, increased destruction. The excessive destruction of platelets is caused by immune mechanisms (e.g. ITP, lupus erythematosus and secondary to drug exposure) or non-immune mechanisms (e.g. pregnancy-induced hypertension (PIH) and disseminated intravascular coagulation (DIC)). The cause may be more serious for the mother or foetus than the thrombocytopaenia itself for example, pre-eclampsia, systemic lupus erythematosus (SLE) and DIC. Haemostasis and foetal risks always need to be assessed when thrombocytopaenia is detected during pregnancy or delivery.

Platelet counts of less than 150×10^9/l have been observed in 7–10% of unselected pregnancies, although severe thrombocytopaenia (platelet count less than 50×10^9/l) is rare, occurring in less than 0.1% of pregnancies. Thrombocytopaenia is usually defined as a platelet count of less than 150×10^9/l, which represents the 2.5th percentile of the distribution in a healthy population of men and non-pregnant

Table 19.1 – Causes of thrombocytopaenia in women.

- Common
  - thrombocytopaenia of pregnancy (GTP) (74%)
  - hypertensive disorders of pregnancy (21%)
  - immune disorders of pregnancy (4%) for example, ITP and SLE
- Uncommon (4%)
  - DIC
  - TTP
  - fatty liver
  - HELLP syndrome
  - antiphospholipid syndrome
- Rare
  - folate deficiency
  - congenital (e.g. May–Hegglin anomaly)
  - hypersplenism
  - coincidental marrow disease

women. A study of 6770 pregnant women near term found the 2.5th percentile for the platelet count at the end of pregnancy was $116 \times 10^9/l$. Thus, in healthy women with no history of thrombocytopaenia, a platelet count of over $115 \times 10^9/l$ late in pregnancy does not require further investigation and is a safe threshold. The causes of thrombocytopaenia during pregnancy are summarised in Table 19.1.

MANAGEMENT OPTIONS AND DISCUSSION

Gestational thrombocytopaenia

Most cases at term are due to gestational thrombocytopaenia (GTP), a benign condition for the mother and foetus, affecting up to 7% of pregnant women. No specific treatment is required. It probably represents an acceleration of the increased platelet destruction during pregnancy. Typically, the thrombocytopaenia is mild to moderate with platelet counts over $70 \times 10^9/l$. When no prior platelet counts are available, GTP cannot be distinguished with certainty from ITP, and the diagnosis depends on follow-up after delivery where the majority of cases resolve quickly, whereas in ITP the condition remains. The differential diagnosis becomes important when treatment is required during pregnancy or at delivery.

Immune thrombocytopenic purpura

This is relatively common during pregnancy, occurring in 1–2/1000 deliveries. Destruction occurs by platelet autoantibodies directed against platelet surface antigens. The course of the disease is not affected by pregnancy but the disease may significantly influence the outcome of pregnancy. There is no reliable confirmatory laboratory test and diagnosis is often by exclusion. Bleeding is less likely at a given platelet count compared to underproduction states, as it is the old platelets that are cleared. This leaves larger than average-sized platelets with increased numbers of platelet granules that have enhance platelet function. The main risk to the mother is haemorrhage during and after childbirth. Factors that aggravate ITP should be avoided, for example, aspirin, alcohol, vaccinations and infection. The goal of management is to achieve a platelet count of over $50 \times 10^9/l$ and corticosteroids are the usual first line treatment. Foetal side effects are unlikely as 90% of a dose of prednisolone is metabolised in the placenta. Maternal side effects are a potential problem, including hypertension, osteoporosis, weight gain, acne and psychosis. Treatment should be monitored and the lowest maintenance dose at which the platelet count remains over $50 \times 10^9/l$ should be selected. If not successful, the duration of therapy is prolonged, or the maintenance dose is unacceptably high, intravenous immunoglobulin can rapidly increase the platelet count. This may be necessary in preparation for Caesarean section, splenectomy, or to treat acute haemorrhage. Splenectomy is possible as a last resort in the second trimester in women with intractable and symptomatic ITP. Immunosuppressive drugs are not suitable in pregnancy due to their teratogenicity. Platelet transfusions are not indicated unless there is life-threatening haemorrhage or a very low platelet count in patients undergoing surgery. Unnecessary platelet transfusions in the absence of haemostatic failure may stimulate more autoantibody production and worsen maternal thrombocytopaenia.

Platelet antibodies (usually IgG) may enter the foetal circulation and cause immune destruction of foetal platelets. An affected foetus may be susceptible to intracranial haemorrhage at birth. However, the risk of serious foetal or neonatal haemorrhage is quite low in women with ITP and current recommendations are to perform delivery by Caesarean section for obstetric indications alone without determining the foetal platelet count. Cord blood should be sampled at delivery and close monitoring for the first few days of life is required.

Pregnancy-induced hypertension

PIH is the second most common cause of thrombocytopaenia in pregnancy. In 15–29%, parturients will show evidence of a consumptive thrombocytopaenia with an additional defect in platelet function. The management is that of pre-eclampsia. Haemolysis, elevated liver enzymes and low platelets (HELLP) syndrome is an extreme variant of pre-eclampsia and is an indication for delivery. Thrombocytopaenia is a prominent feature and may be severe with platelet counts below $50 \times 10^9/l$. Inadequate haemostasis or excess bleeding is common and blood, fresh frozen plasma and/or platelet transfusions are often required. Thrombocytopaenia seen in severe pre-eclampsia may be secondary to DIC.

Thrombotic thrombocytopenic purpura

TTP is rare, but progression is often rapid and fatal. It is characterised by thrombocytopaenia, haemolytic anaemia, neurological dysfunction, renal failure and fever.

The pathology is widespread with thrombotic occlusion of arterioles and capillaries involving multiple organs. It is important to differentiate TTP from severe PIH or HELLP because the latter are strong indications for delivery, whereas there is no evidence that delivery affects the course of TTP. However, if presenting late in pregnancy, delivery allows aggressive treatment of the mother without risk to the foetus. The main treatment is plasma exchange, usually combined with corticosteroids. Antiplatelet drugs have also been used. Haemolytic uraemic syndrome (HUS) is a related condition usually occurring postpartum with the primary pathology confined to the kidneys.

Drug-induced thrombocytopaenia

Thrombocytopaenia may be secondary to drugs, such as heparin, quinine, penicillins, thiazides, hydralazine, H_2-receptor antagonists, digoxin and cocaine. Bleeding manifestations develop within 24 h of drug exposure and disappear 3–4 days after drug withdrawal. Some drug reactions are peculiar to pregnancy for example, cocaine may cause an acute thrombocytopaenia within hours of use and platelet counts can drop dramatically over the ensuing week without further re-exposure to the drug. Thiazides and hydralazine used by the mother may cause a neonatal thrombocytopaenia.

Anaesthetic management

The main dilemma for anaesthetists is whether regional anaesthesia (RA) is safe for a patient with thrombocytopaenia. The decision depends on the degree of thrombocytopaenia and its aetiology. To determine the cause, a thorough history is required, especially of medications taken and a family or personal history of easy bruising or bleeding. A targeted physical examination to include petechiae, eccymoses, oedema, abdominal and neurology signs should be carried out. Laboratory tests should include full blood count, blood film, coagulation screen, electrolytes and liver function tests. Generally, if the platelets are less than $50 \times 10^9/l$, RA is contraindicated; if the count is over $100 \times 10^9/l$ RA is considered safe. Platelet counts between $50–100 \times 10^9/l$ cause the most concern and have to be considered on an individual basis, as opinions vary as to the lower acceptable limit for platelet count and the performance of RA. Recent opinions have argued for a lower safe limit of $75 \times 10^9/l$ and even $50 \times 10^9/l$ as long as the platelet function is normal and there is no history of bleeding as in GTP and ITP.

In PIH, platelet function may be impaired and a test of platelet function is ideally required. The bleeding time is not reliable. Some centres use thromboelastography, although this is not widely available. The platelet count may fall rapidly (e.g. HELLP syndrome) and the speed of descent may be too fast to safely initiate RA, and bleeding manifestations may be present. All patients require an individual risk/benefit analysis of RA. If the decision favours RA, experienced operators should perform the block, and spinal is preferable to epidural anaesthesia because of the smaller needle. If an epidural is required, a flexible catheter is less traumatic. Removal of the epidural catheter needs to be judged according to the clinical picture. Post-partum monitoring of neurological function is essential to detect early signs of bleeding in the epidural space. In addition, it is wise to avoid drugs that impair platelet function (e.g. aspirin) and non-steroidal anti-inflammatory drugs as well as intramuscular injections.

KEY LEARNING POINTS

1. Thrombocytopaenia in pregnancy is relatively common and unnec-essary investigations are to be avoided in the majority of cases.

2. Severe thrombocytopaenia has risks to the mother and foetus of haemorrhage at delivery and needs thorough investigation and treatment.

3. When considering the safety of RA, the platelet function as well as the absolute level of platelet count is relevant. Other important fac-tors are the aetiology of the thrombocytopaenia and the stability of the platelet count.

4. A careful history and examination for petechiae and bruising is important as a measure of platelet function and coagulopathy.

Further reading

Beilin Y, Zahn J, Comerford M. Safe epidural analgesia in thirty parturients with platelet counts between 69,000 and 98,000 mm^{-3}. *Anesthesia and Analgesia* 1997; **85**: 385–8.

Biswas A, Arulkumaran S, Ratnam SS. Disorders of platelets in pregnancy. *Obstetrical and Gynecological Survey* 1994; **49**: 585–94.

Boehlen F, Hohlfeld P, Extermann P, Perneger TV, De Moerloose P. Platelet count at term pregnancy: a reappraisal of the threshold. *Obstetrics and Gynecology* 2000; **95**: 29–33.

Burrows RF, Kelton JG. Pregnancy in patients with idiopathic thrombocytopenic purpura: assessing the risks for the infant at delivery. *Obstetrical and Gynecological Survey* 1993; **48**: 781–8.

Burrows RF, Kelton JG. Fetal thrombocytopaenia and its relation to maternal thrombocytopaenia. *The New England Journal of Medicine* 1993; **329**: 1463–6.

Douglas MJ. Platelets, the parturient and regional anesthesia. *International Journal of Obstetric Anesthesia* 2001; **10**: 113–20.

Hawthorne L. Haematological disorders in pregnancy. In: Russell IF and Lyons G (eds) *Clinical Problems in Obstetric Anaesthesia*. Chapman and Hall, London, 1997, pp. 67–84.

Letsky EA, Greaves M. Guidelines on the investigation and management of thrombocytopaenia in pregnancy and neonatal alloimmune thrombocyto-paenia. *British Journal of Haematology* 1996; **95**: 21–6.

Sainio S, Kekomaki R, Riikonen S, Teramo K. Maternal thrombocytopaenia at term: a population-based study. *Acta Obstetricia et Gynecologica Scandinavica* 2000; **79**: 744–9.

Shehata N, Burrows R, Kelton JG. Gestational thrombocytopenia. *Clinical Obstetrics and Gynecology* 1999; **42**: 327–34.

Silver RM, Ware Branch D, Scott JR. Maternal thrombocytopaenia in pregnancy: time for a reassessment. *American Journal of Obstetrics and Gynecology* 1995; **173**: 479–82.

INDEX

abdominal compression, in post-dural
  puncture headache 125
abscesses, in injecting drug users 47–48
accidental dural puncture (ADP) 121,
  122–123
  after previous spinal surgery 147
  incidence 122
  management 124–125 (Table)
  prevention 124
ACTH (adrenocorticotrophic hormone)
  121, 126
activated partial thromboplastin time
  (APTT) 5–6
acute renal failure, in pre-eclampsia 137
acute tubular necrosis 137
aggressive behaviour, drug abusers 45
airway
  fibre-optic assessment 87
  intubation *see* intubation, tracheal
  management, in pre-eclampsia/eclampsia
    140–141
  oedema, in pre-eclampsia 136, 140
alfentanil, in emergency Caesarean
    section 32
allergy, latex 91–96
amino-caproic acid 76
aminophylline 10, 11, 14–15
amniotic fluid, in salvaged blood 77
amniotic fluid embolism (AFE) 77
amphetamine abuse 50
anaemia
  antenatal management 75
  in Jehovah's Witness 71
  pathophysiology 74
anaesthetist, delay in attending 97–98,
    99–100
analgesia for labour

in asthma 16
in breech delivery 19–20, 21–23
in drug abuse 51
in pre-eclampsia 140
anaphylactic reaction, latex 93
ante-partum haemorrhage (APH) 55, 58
antibiotic treatment, legal aspects 98, 100,
    101, 103
anticholinergics, inhaled 15
anticoagulation
  regional anaesthesia and 1–8
  surgery in diabetic pregnancy and 36, 41
antihypertensive therapy
  in diabetic pregnancy 35, 37, 40
  in pre-eclampsia 133–134 (Table),
    135 (Fig.)
aortocaval compression 28–29
  prevention 15, 32
aprotinin 60, 76
aspiration, gastric 28
  prevention 15, 30–32
aspirin, regional anaesthesia and 1, 4
asthma 9–18
  acute severe 9–11, 12, 13–16
  assessment of severity 12 (Table)
  maternal and foetal complications 12–13
attitudes
  to drug abusers 51
  to Jehovah's Witnesses 74–75
autonomic nervous system, in
    pre-eclampsia 132
autonomic neuropathy, diabetic 35, 41
awake intubation 88, 155
azathioprine 115

back pain, after previous spinal surgery 145,
    148–149